Protecting the Future

HIV Prevention, Care, and Support
Among Displaced and War-Affected Populations

WENDY HOLMES, MB BS MSc
for the International Rescue Committee

Illustrations by Julie Smith

IRC

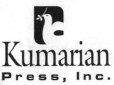
Kumarian
Press, Inc.

Protecting the Future: HIV Prevention, Care, and Support Among Displaced and War-Affected Populations

Published 2003 in the United States of America by Kumarian Press, Inc.
1294 Blue Hills Avenue, Bloomfield, CT 06002 USA.

Exclusive distributor for Europe and nonexclusive distributor for the rest of the world excluding the USA and Canada: Oxfam Publishing, Oxfam GB, 274 Banbury Road, Oxford, OX2 7DZ, UK.

Production, design, indexing, and proofreading
by ediType, Yorktown Heights, New York

The text of this book is set in 11/13 Adobe Sabon.

Printed in the United States on acid-free paper by Thomson-Shore, Inc.
Text printed with vegetable oil–based ink.

♾ The paper used in this publication meets the minimum requirements of the American National Standard for Information Sciences–Permanence of Paper for Printed Library Materials, ANSI Z39.48-1984.

Library of Congress Cataloging-in-Publication Data

Holmes, Wendy, 1956-
    Protecting the future : HIV prevention, care, and support among
displaced and war-affected populations / Wendy Holmes ; illustrations by
Julie Smith.
      p. ; cm.
    Includes bibliographical references and index.
    ISBN 1-56549-162-9 (pbk. : alk. paper)
    1. AIDS (Disease) – Prevention. 2. AIDS (Disease) – Patients – Services
for. 3. Non-governmental organizations. 4. Refugees – Medical care.
[DNLM: 1. HIV Infections – prevention & control. 2. Community Health
Services – organization & administration. WC 503.6 H753p 2003]
I. Title.
RA643.8.H65 2003
616.97'9205 – dc21

                                2003001618

---

12 11 10 09 08 07 06 05 04 03   10 9 8 7 6 5 4 3 2 1   First Printing 2003

Contents

Acknowledgements   vii

Abbreviations   ix

Introduction: Why Humanitarian
Agencies Should Concern Themselves
with HIV Prevention and Care   1

Part 1
PREPARING YOURSELVES

1. Exploring Your Own Knowledge,
Attitudes, and Behavior   9

2. Basic Facts about HIV Infection   19

3. Thinking about the Communities
You Work With   29

4. What Role Might NGOs Play in
the Response to HIV?   33

Part 2
ENGAGING THE COMMUNITY

5. Gathering Information —
Analyzing the Situation   37

6. The Strategic Planning Process   55

Part 3
WHAT CAN WE DO TO CONTRIBUTE
TO HIV PREVENTION AND CARE?

7. Counseling for HIV Prevention
and Care   67

8. Preventing Transmission through Sex   83

9. Strategies for Prevention of
Transmission through Injecting
Drug Use   123

10. Enabling People to Live Positively
with HIV   131

Part 4
ISSUES FOR
HEALTH CARE SERVICES

11. Prevention and Care in Relation
to Parent-to-Child Transmission   139

12. Prevention of Transmission
through Blood Transfusion   159

13. Prevention of Transmission in
Health Care Settings   167

14. Providing Care and Support   175

Appendix A: Questions to Assist
in Planning a Situation Analysis   193

Appendix B: HIV Testing Strategies   199

Appendix C: PLA Exercises for
Gathering Sensitive Information —
Some Examples   201

Appendix D: Syndromic Management
of Sexually Transmitted Infections   207

Appendix E: Selected References,
Resources, and Further Reading   215

Index   219

Acknowledgments

This manual was prepared following consultation with the staff of the International Rescue Committee (IRC) in New York and with IRC field staff in Rwanda, Democratic Republic of Congo, Tanzania, Macedonia, and Albania in November 2000. I would like to thank the IRC Country Directors, Health Coordinators, and their teams for sharing their experiences with me, for discussing their ideas in relation to HIV prevention and care in the settings where they work, and for their warm hospitality.

I am grateful to Rich Brennan, Mary Otieno, Sandra Krause, and Lisa Sherburne for their advice and support. I would also like to thank Karla Meursing, Kim Benton, Bev Snell, Mike Toole, Tamara Kwarteng, Michelle Kermode, Trish Clark, and Chris Goethel for their contributions and comments. Thanks to Julie Smith for the illustrations.

The development of the manual was funded through the generous support of the Bill and Melinda Gates Foundation.

Wendy Holmes
Macfarlane Burnet Institute for
Medical Research and Public Health
Melbourne, November 2001

Abbreviations

AIDS	Acquired Immune Deficiency Syndrome
ARVP	Antiretroviral prophylaxis
ARVs	Antiretroviral (anti-HIV) drugs
AZT	Zidovudine (an antiretroviral drug)
CDC	U.S. Centers for Disease Control and Prevention (Atlanta)
DNA	Deoxyribonucleic acid (genetic instructions in a cell)
ELISA	Enzyme-Linked Immunosorbent Assay (HIV antibody test)
FGD	Focus group discussion
HIV	Human Immunodeficiency Virus
IDP	Internally displaced person
IEC	Information, Education, Communication
IRC	International Rescue Committee
MCH	Maternal and child health
MISP	Minimum Initial Service Package
MTCT	Mother-to-child transmission
NGOs	Non-governmental organizations
NNRTIs	Non-nucleoside reverse transcriptase inhibitors (antiretroviral drug)
NRTIs	Nucleoside reverse transcriptase inhibitors (antiretroviral drug)
PCR	Polymerase chain reaction (test for HIV)
PEP	Post-exposure prophylaxis
PIs	Protease inhibitors (antiretroviral drug)
PLA	Participatory learning and action
PLWH	People/person living with HIV/AIDS. Also PLWH/A
PTCT	Parent-to-child transmission
SGBV	Sexual and gender-based violence
SIV	Simian (monkey) immunodeficiency virus
STI	Sexually transmitted infection
TASO	The AIDS Support Organisation (Uganda)
TB	Tuberculosis

UNAIDS	Joint United Nations Programme on HIV/AIDS
UNDP	United Nations Development Programme
UNFPA	United Nations Population Fund
UNHCR	United Nations High Commissioner for Refugees
UNICEF	United Nations Children's Fund
VCT	Voluntary counseling and testing
WB	Western blot (confirmatory HIV antibody test)
WHO	World Health Organization

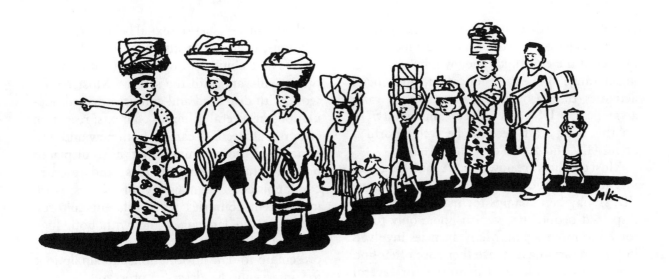

Introduction

Why Humanitarian Agencies Should Concern Themselves with HIV Prevention and Care

We know that when populations move in large numbers because of a crisis they are vulnerable to the rapid spread of infections: to cholera, other diarrheal diseases, measles, and malaria. Sexually transmitted infections (STIs), including HIV, also spread quickly among displaced populations. In crisis situations women and men are often subjected to sexual assaults and may have to exchange sex for money or food to survive. Blood may be transfused without screening. Normal patterns of sexual behavior are often disrupted, and young people may have sex more often and with more partners than they would in their usual circumstances. Local or international military and the host population may be interacting sexually with the displaced population and may have higher rates of STIs and HIV. The purpose of providing clean water, food, shelter, measles vaccination,

and malaria control is defeated if the lives saved are later lost to AIDS.

The HIV epidemic presents a challenge to humanitarian agencies both in the acute emergency phase and afterward. During the acute emergency phase it is essential to provide easy access to condoms, to screen blood for transfusion for HIV, and to protect vulnerable populations from rape. Once the situation is more stable humanitarian agencies can work with their beneficiaries to develop community-based strategies to minimize further spread of HIV and provide care and support to those affected.

Humanitarian agencies that have been present during a crisis will be in a useful position to undertake such work. They may have gained the trust of the refugees/IDPs and local population. They may have established good communication with the host government and therefore

1

be able to advocate for effective and appropriate strategies to prevent HIV and modify the impact of the epidemic. They will be establishing a range of health, education, and social activities that provide opportunities to raise awareness of HIV and reduce vulnerability. To do this their staff need to be well informed about HIV and aware of its importance.

Most conflicts are now complex and long lasting. Refugees and internally displaced persons (IDPs) may be in camps for many years; these displaced people may return home only to be forced to move again. Many agencies involved in humanitarian assistance therefore often find themselves remaining in countries for several years. After the period of crisis there is a need for a more community-based, development-oriented approach. For this changed role staff need to have different skills and experience from those needed during a crisis, when water, sanitation, food, and shelter are the priorities. Development activities are also influenced by the uncertain, artificial, and temporary nature of refugees' and IDPs' lives, especially in camps.

In recent years there has been a new emphasis on the reproductive health needs and concerns of refugees and IDPs, and on the problem of sexual and gender-based violence. A great deal has already been learned and documented about how to tackle these sensitive issues. This experience is of great relevance to HIV prevention and care.

In some countries the impact of the HIV epidemic has been disastrous. Non-governmental organizations (NGOs) have a role in helping communities to prepare for disasters associated with large movements of refugees and IDPs. It is also appropriate to assist people to prepare for and prevent the slow disaster of the HIV epidemic.

CHALLENGES TO INCORPORATING HIV PREVENTION, CARE, AND SUPPORT IN SETTINGS OF DISPLACEMENT AND CONFLICT

Addressing HIV in different contexts

Successful interventions in relation to HIV prevention and care are built on an understanding of the sensitive issues of sexual behavior, gender relations, drug use, health care, and dying, as well as on technical knowledge. What is appropriate will vary with the setting. Most NGOs work with displaced and conflict-affected populations in several different contexts: reception centers; refugee/IDP camps, both new and well established; communities that host displaced people; refugee-impacted areas; and resettled communities. The majority of NGOs work in different countries with different cultures, histories, and languages and with both high and low HIV prevalence. In this manual we present up-to-date information, explain options for interventions, describe processes, suggest ideas, describe experiences, and point the way to additional resources. We hope that this will assist NGO staff to gather information, prioritize interventions, and implement activities that will be appropriate for their context. The manual is designed primarily for the late-emergency and post-emergency phases of complex emergencies. The UNAIDS document *Guidelines for HIV Interventions in Emergency Settings* is a useful resource for the acute emergency phase.

The manual should also be a useful resource for those working toward the reconstruction of health care service systems in the aftermath of conflict; it is important to build in HIV prevention and care efforts from the start.

Integrating HIV prevention and care with existing activities

It is important that a manual on HIV prevention and care guidelines does not lead to the development of separate HIV projects in refugee/IDP camps or affected communities. Awareness of the risk of spread of HIV among refugees, internally displaced, and other conflict-affected populations is growing. Donors may call for proposals that address this issue. But when preparing a proposal for HIV prevention and care activities it is important to think about how these will be integrated with existing activities.

Even for refugees and IDPs who are aware of HIV, the threat of a disease that may kill them in years to come is not likely to be a priority when they are struggling to survive or fatalistic about the future. However, unwanted pregnancy, STIs, and resulting infertility are often of great concern to them. There may not be a need to specifically focus on HIV control in these settings because activities that promote sexual health and prevent STIs and unwanted pregnancy will also reduce the risk of spread of HIV.

Often a great deal is already being done that contributes to the prevention of spread of HIV. This needs to be recognized. For example:

- projects that aim to increase the skills and confidence of young people can assist them to better protect themselves from unsafe sex;

- in general, promotion of exclusive breast-feeding will help to reduce the risk of transmission of HIV to babies in populations when it is not known which women are infected;

- income-generating activities for women may help them to avoid hazardous sex work; and

- efforts to protect women from sexual violence also protect them from HIV.

The manual includes stories of relevant activities carried out in different humanitarian settings.

An HIV prevention and care component can often be added to existing activities.

- HIV and STI information can be a theme within projects for young people — as the topic for a play or a poster competition.

- Booklets on aspects of HIV infection can be used in literacy programs.

- There may be the opportunity for community health workers undertaking home visits to provide one-to-one education about HIV, identify and arrange treatment for STIs, and distribute condoms.

"Primary health care," "reproductive health," "maternal health," "sexual and gender-based violence," "family planning," and "HIV/AIDS" are overlapping categories. It is important not to develop separate programs in these areas, but

to integrate activities, including the training of counselors.

It is also important that focusing on reproductive health and HIV prevention does not divert resources away from other necessary life-saving measures.

Coordinating and collaborating with other sectors

At the government level HIV prevention and care efforts are usually coordinated and funded through the ministry of health. However, it is widely recognized that the factors that increase the spread of HIV concern many sectors of society, and the impact of the epidemic is broad. The response to HIV needs to be intersectoral. It is important that this manual is not used only by health professionals, but also by staff working in education, welfare, and children and youth programs, and with sexual and gender-based violence issues.

Addressing controversial issues

Planning HIV prevention and care interventions raises many controversial issues. Some behaviors and practices that increase the risk of spread of HIV may be illegal and/or stigmatized, such as sex work, injecting drug use, sex before or outside marriage, and homosexuality. Strategies to promote modifications of these behaviors in order to reduce the risk of the spread of HIV may be seen by some to condone the behaviors. Within the manual we present a number of boxes containing "Discussion points" to help guide group discussions. Health staff may have their own concerns about exposure to the virus; some staff may be infected. The manual emphasizes the importance of initial awareness raising and training for all staff, and suggests ways to explore attitudes and promote a nonjudgmental and nondiscriminatory approach.

Developing an ethical and human rights framework

Much progress has been made in recent years in linking the fields of public health and human rights. Too often strategies to prevent the spread of HIV aim to alter the behavior of individuals and fail to take into account sufficiently the societal factors that determine vulnerability. A human rights framework can help to generate new creative approaches to address the spread and impact of HIV.

When planning and implementing HIV prevention and care work there are ethical issues to consider in relation to:

- gathering quantitative and qualitative information,

- surveillance,

- blood screening,

- establishing voluntary counseling and testing services, and

- preventing mother-to-child transmission of HIV.

These ethical issues are explored in the relevant sections of the manual, with suggestions for ways to avoid causing unintended harm.

Understanding gender analysis

In planning to address the problem of HIV it is important to understand the roles, responsibilities, and rights of men and of women, and the relationships between them. Men and women are different and play different roles in all societies, but should share equal rights and status. We need to recognize that gender roles and relationships are often changed as a result of crises, especially when refugees/IDPs live for a long time in camp settings. Gender analysis involves thinking about the impact of activities on gender roles and on gender equity.

Involving men

Because women more often suffer the consequences of poor reproductive health, they are often the focus of attention in reproductive health programs. However, the reproductive health status of men has a direct effect on that of women. Many HIV interventions have failed because they have not engaged men. It is essential to consider the knowledge, attitudes, and behaviors of men as well as women, and to engage men in HIV prevention and care.

Using resources

A great deal has already been learned about effective ways to respond to the HIV epidemic. It is important to learn from the experiences of others. There are many existing sources of information, resources, and training materials. Indeed there are so many materials available on HIV, in journals and books and on the Internet, that it easy to become confused. We have identified a small range of particularly useful resources to form a mini-library on HIV/AIDS for staff. There are lists of additional resources at the end of chapters and an annotated list of resources and addresses in appendix E (page 215). If you cannot access the Internet ask staff at headquarters to obtain the information you need. The manual also includes a range of sample checklists and guidelines for different situations.

This manual aims to supplement the 1999 *Reproductive Health in Refugee Situations Field Manual,* which has been widely used.

Coping with constraints and frustrations

NGO staff live and work in difficult conditions. There is always too much to do, too little time, and too few resources. With competing demands it is difficult to address the spread of HIV. Interventions often concern numerous stakeholders with different points of view, and the technical issues can be difficult to understand. It is not easy to persuade people to change their behavior. In this manual we try to acknowledge the limitations workers face and the frustrations that occur. We try to avoid telling you what you should do and instead make suggestions and give ideas.

We hope that this manual will assist you to achieve your mission of improving the social, economic, and health status of refugees/IDPs and victims of oppression or violent conflict.

HOW TO USE THIS MANUAL

The manual may be used in a number of ways:

- to find suggestions for ways to integrate HIV prevention and care activities with the work that you and your team are already doing;

- to assist in planning and proposal writing for new HIV prevention and care activities;

- as a reference to check information or to point the way to other relevant resources. HIV is a rapidly changing area; the resources mentioned can help in staying up to date;

- as a source of ideas for training exercises. Although this is not a training manual, there are examples of games, exercises, and discussion points that can be useful in teaching, raising awareness, and planning;

- to help in orientation for new staff;

- to find and photocopy checklists and guidelines that you can use or adapt for your own programs and settings.

HOW THE MANUAL IS ORGANIZED

Part 1: Preparing yourselves

Part 1 is about preparing yourself and your team. It includes ideas to stimulate discussion and explore attitudes. It provides some basic up-to-date information about HIV infection and answers some of the questions most frequently asked by field staff. Then there are some suggestions for how to identify ways to integrate HIV prevention and care activities with existing activities.

Part 2: Engaging the community

Part 2 deals with how to engage the local community. Different settings require different strategies. There will always be a need to gather information in a participatory way to inform local strategic planning, to consult closely with local stakeholders, and to engage community members in the response to the epidemic.

Part 3: What can we do to contribute to HIV prevention and care?

Part 3 presents information about strategies and interventions that contribute to HIV prevention and care. Each chapter has an *introduction* to describe the strategy; a *rationale*, which presents the arguments and evidence for adopting the approach; a description of some possible *strategies*; some examples of appropriate evaluation *indicators* and some suggested *additional resources*. This manual does not include instructions for proposal writing or project design,* but we hope that this structure will be useful when preparing funding proposals.

Part 4: Issues for health care services

Although the response to the epidemic needs to be intersectoral, there are some issues that are inevitably the concern of health care services, so we have placed these in one part. Among these issues are prevention of the spread of the virus from mother to child, through blood transfusions, and in clinics and hospitals. The continuum of care needs to extend to home-based care in the community, but since this is most likely to be coordinated by health care services, we have also included the issue of providing care, and looking after the carers, in this part.

Appendices

The appendices contain lists of resources and useful addresses, question guides and ideas for participatory exercises useful for information gathering, and reference material in relation to HIV testing strategies and management protocols for STIs.

---

*For this see, for example, *The Training Guide to IRC's Program Design, Monitoring, and Evaluation Framework,* International Rescue Committee and Columbia University, Joseph L. Mailman, School of Public Health, New York, 2000, and *IRC's Proposal Guidelines Based on the Causal Pathway.*

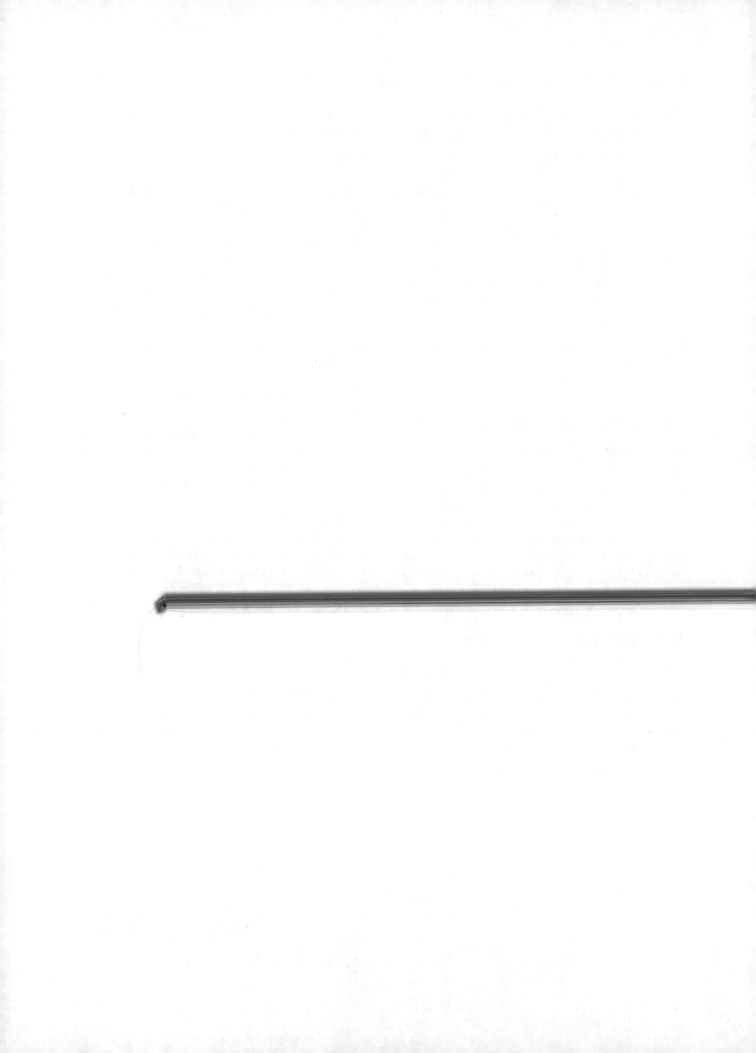

Part 1

PREPARING YOURSELVES

The first step in planning how to incorporate HIV prevention and care is to raise awareness within your own team. Think about whether you need to include others that you work closely with, such as other NGOs or local government counterparts, at this early stage. Of course consultation with all stakeholders is essential, but it is important to prepare for this first.

You may already be undertaking HIV-related activities — but you may still like to hold one or more sessions with all the staff to make sure that all are aware and have up-to-date knowledge.

In these sessions you might aim to:

- check understanding and increase people's knowledge of HIV infection;

- answer any questions and correct common misconceptions;

- provide an opportunity for staff to explore their own attitudes and beliefs;

- think about the characteristics of the population that you work with in order to identify:

  - factors that make them vulnerable to HIV

  - strengths that may help them to protect themselves and to care for those infected, and

  - the likely impact of the epidemic

- gather ideas for incorporating HIV prevention and care activities into your existing activities.

In part 1 we present some ideas on how to do this, the basic facts about HIV/AIDS, and answers to some commonly asked questions.

If you will be the facilitator for these sessions we suggest that you read through chapter 2 ("Basic Facts about HIV Infection") and the answers to the "commonly asked questions" (page 25) before the session.

1

Exploring Your Own Knowledge, Attitudes, and Behavior

NGO staff come from a variety of backgrounds, cultures, and religions and have different beliefs and attitudes. Staff often work under stressful conditions. It is important to acknowledge this and to think about possible implications for HIV prevention and care work.

Some staff may be worried about their own risk of HIV infection, and some may know that they are infected but not wish to disclose this. Take care to avoid an "us and them" tone in the discussions.

In some societies there will be an expectation that unmarried staff have no sexual experience. These staff may then feel uncomfortable discussing sexual health and sexual practices. Staff with certain religious beliefs may not be willing to promote or discuss safer sexual practices such as mutual masturbation, interfemoral sex (sex between the thighs), or condom use because they believe the practices are immoral.

In most societies it is not culturally acceptable to talk openly about sex, especially with members of the opposite sex. It is important to begin by pointing this out and explaining that because of the spread of HIV and STIs it is important for our work that we know about and feel comfortable to discuss a wide variety of sexual behaviors, attitudes, and practices. But sex is an interesting subject, and it is often surprising how willing people are to talk about sex when they are given "permission."

Take into account that staff may have different cultural expectations of the roles of men and women and of what behavior is appropriate for the different sexes and between sexes. In this environment it is easy for misunderstandings and problems to occur. With discussion such problems can often be prevented, but arrangements need to be available to manage problems in the workplace, including sexual harassment, if they do occur. It is helpful to nominate a male and a female person whom staff know that they can talk to in confidence if they experience a problem with another staff member.

The number of information and discussion sessions to have will depend on the experience and knowledge of the team, but it is sensible to have at least two because the first session may raise questions or issues that can be addressed at the second session. A good way to begin a session is with a game or exercise, such as one of those that follow, which allow participants to check their knowledge and to start to talk about sensitive topics.

TRANSMISSION PICTURE CARD GAME

Materials

Two sets of five cards with "No risk, "Very low risk," "Low risk," "Medium risk," and "High risk" written on them.

There are two sets of picture cards (pages 11 and 12), which you can photocopy and adapt as necessary. Cut out the pictures and stick them on cardboard. If you have time you can color the pictures and laminate them so that you have a long-lasting resource for HIV training.

Instructions

- On each of two tables, or on the floor, lay out the "risk" cards.

- Divide the participants into two teams, and give each team a set of sixteen picture cards.

- Ask the participants to discuss each behavior or situation shown on the cards to decide in which risk category the card belongs.

- When they have finished each team should look at the other's table to see whether they agree.

Participants may argue about what the words "high risk" and "low risk" mean. This is a useful discussion. Explain that in real life there are no clear-cut categories of risk—but rather a transition from low to high risk.

In discussing the picture that represents sexual intercourse they may say that they cannot decide about the level of risk because they do not know whether one of the sex partners is infected with HIV. You can point out that this is true in real life.

You might introduce the idea of "attributable risk" — how many of the total number of cases of HIV infection can be attributed to a particular risk factor? For example, a single act of vaginal sexual intercourse between a couple where one has HIV carries a low risk of transmission if both partners have healthy genitals. Yet heterosexual sex is undoubtedly the most common route of the spread of HIV in the world. It is a common behavior, frequently repeated. If a blood transfusion of HIV-infected blood is given to a patient the risk of transmission is 100 percent, but this event happens less often.

Participants may also have a useful discussion about the picture of the whisky bottle. HIV does not spread through drinking alcohol or sharing glasses, but drinking may lead to unwise decisions in relation to unprotected sex or needle sharing.

Summarize the discussion at the end of the game, and have a break.

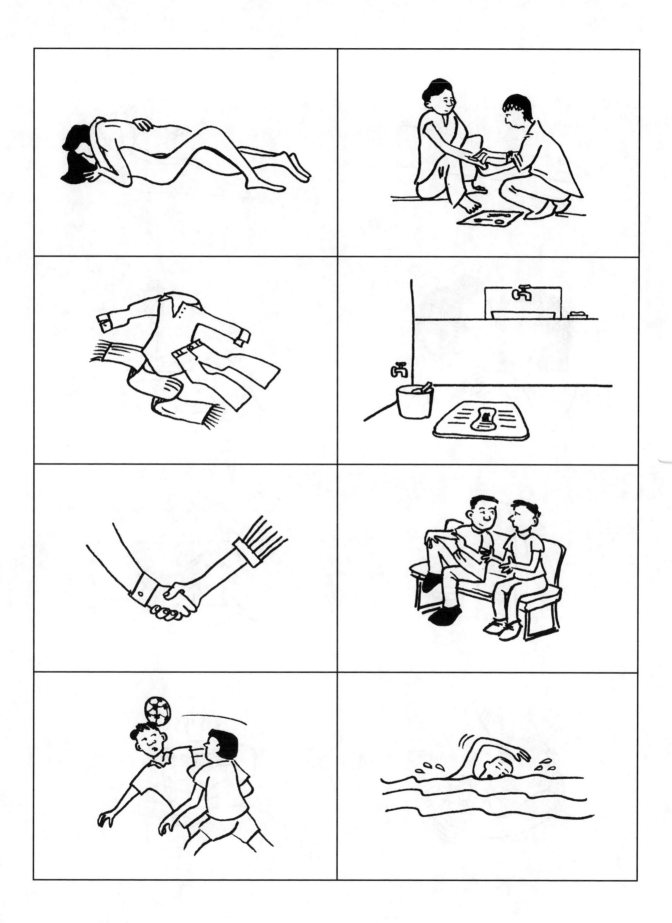

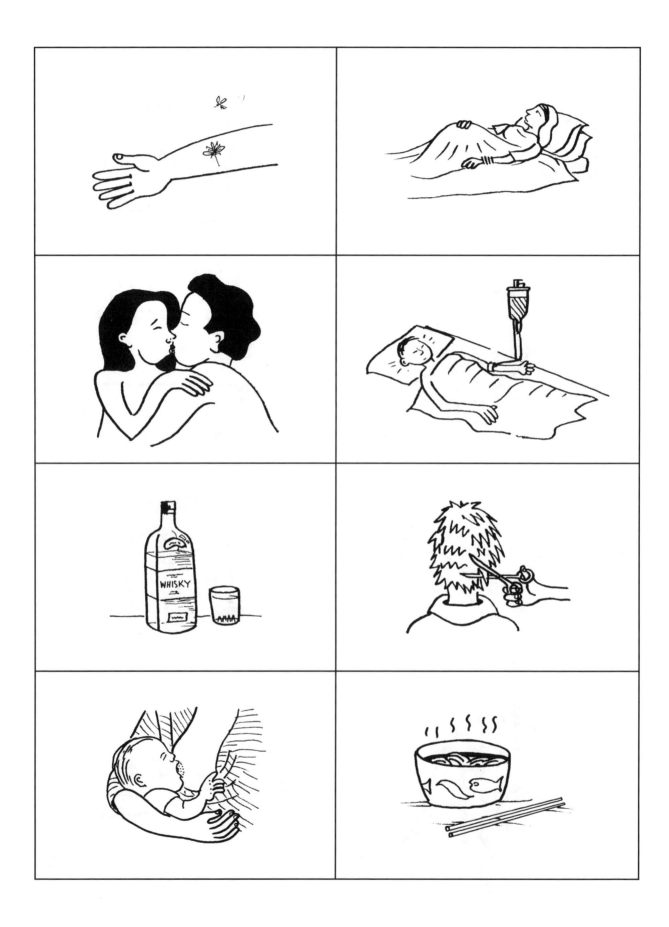

HIV EPIDEMIC EXERCISE

Materials

- One white cup for each participant
- Enough water to fill each cup one-third full
- Enough starch solution to fill one or two cups one-third full
- 10 ml of polyvidone iodine 10 percent
- An "instruction" card for each participant
- Pens to write on the cups

Preparation before the exercise

Instruction cards: On one or two cards write: "Mix your water with ten or more other people's water." If you have twenty participants or less, make one card with these instructions; if more than twenty make two.

On half of the remaining cards write: "Mix your water with four or five different people's water."

On half the remaining cards write: "Mix your water with one other person's water. Do this with the same person four times."

On the rest of the cards write: "Touch your glass with the glass of two or three other people. Do not mix your water with anyone."

Starch solution: Make the starch solution by mixing half a teaspoon of clothes starch (or maize flour or cassava flour) in a cup that is one-third full of water (or water that has been used to cook rice). If you use flour instead of starch, or rice water instead of water, test that the exercise will work before the lesson.

Before the participants arrive, fill one cup only one-third full with starch solution. If you have more than twenty participants, fill two cups one-third with starch solution. Fill all other cups one-third full with water. You may need to add a few drops of milk to the water to make it look the same as the starch solution. If the solution in the cups containing the starch looks a bit cloudy, then add a few drops of milk to the glasses of plain water so that all the cups look the same.

Instructions

Introduce the exercise by explaining that the purpose is to show how rapidly HIV can spread. Explain that in this exercise mixing the water in your glass represents the sharing of body fluids that occurs during sex. Touching glasses together without mixing the water represents using a condom during sex. Explain that in the exercise, as in life, there will be some people who "have sex" with many people, and some who "have sex" with only one person. A few use condoms, but most don't. The instruction cards will tell them which role to play. Do not mention that one of the cups is different from the others.

—Adapted from "Wildfire," First Caribbean HIV and Development Workshop, *Facilitators' Workbook,* 1999, *www.undp.org,* and an exercise in K. Birrell and G. Birrell, *Diagnosis and Treatment: A Training Manual for Primary Health Care Workers* (Macmillan Education Ltd., 2000).

HIV EPIDEMIC EXERCISE (CONTINUED)

Although this exercise usually leads to a lot of laughter, remember that some participants may feel awkward or embarrassed when they take part. Also, bear in mind that one or more participants may in fact be infected with HIV. Explain that although the exercise is fun, it has a serious purpose.

Hold the cards so that you cannot see the instructions, but make sure that you have one that says "Mix your water with ten or more other people's water" on the top. Give one participant the cup with the starch solution (which looks just the same as the other cups) and the top instruction card. Give all other participants cups with water and a card.

Next ask the participants to walk around the room and talk to at least four other participants. Tell them, "If your card and the card of the person you are talking to tells you to mix water together, pour your water into the other cup and then pour half back into your own cup."

After ten to fifteen minutes ask the participants to stop. Say, "Now it is three months later. You have all been counseled and decided that you would like to have an HIV test. In this exercise we represent the HIV blood test by adding drops of iodine to the water in your cup. If the water turns blue this represents a positive test result. If the water turns yellow or brown, this represents a negative result. To preserve confidentiality before you send your sample to the lab for testing please put a four-letter or four-digit code, which you will remember, on the cup."

Then ask the participants to put their cards face down on the table with the cup on top. Put four drops of polyvidone iodine 10 percent into each cup. Tell everyone how many of the cups have turned blue (i.e., tested positive). Ask them to calculate what percentage this is. Read out some of the instruction cards for the positive cups and some for the negative cups. Next call out the code numbers and give the participants their cups so that they can see their "result."

Tell the participants that at the beginning of the exercise only one person was "infected with HIV." Ask if anyone knew who was "infected" before the exercise.

Finally ask all the participants what we can learn from this exercise. They may make some of the following points:

- Most people with HIV do not know that they are infected. They may infect a large number of other people without knowing.

- It is not possible to know from looking at a person whether that person is infected with HIV or not.

- Condoms protect against HIV infection.

- If a person has only one sexual partner, that person may still become infected with HIV if the partner has other sexual partners.

- People who have many sexual partners and who do not use condoms are most likely to become infected with HIV.

- The time of waiting for the HIV test result is likely to be a worrying time for people, especially if they have to keep it secret.

GROUP DISCUSSION EXERCISE: TALKING ABOUT GENDER EXPECTATIONS

This is a useful and nonthreatening session that works well with a mixed group of men and women from different backgrounds.

Ask members of the group to think of rhymes or proverbs that they were taught as children and that carried messages about what boys and girls, or men and women, should be like. An example from British culture is:

Sugar and spice and all things nice, that's what little girls are made of.
Rats and snails and puppy dog tails, that's what little boys are made of.

This often leads to a discussion about what the "real" innate differences are between the sexes and what differences are the result of society's expectations. Did society's expectations come from observations of innate gender differences? It may also lead to a discussion about how those who do not fit into gender stereotypes feel — and what reactions they trigger from other people.

If you have time you can finish the discussion by asking what might be the implications for HIV prevention.

GROUP DISCUSSION EXERCISE: TALKING ABOUT SEXUALITY AND SEXUAL HEALTH

First introduce the exercise. "This morning we are going to talk about sex. Sex is always an interesting topic. In most societies there are taboos and unwritten rules about discussing sex. We have to agree today that although it is not usual to discuss sex in detail, we are professionals who want to prevent the spread of STIs and HIV and to promote sexual health, so we need to be able to talk about sexual matters."

Ask the participants to break into smaller groups of three or four and discuss the following questions in relation to their own society:

- Is it easy to talk about sex? Is this different for men and for women, for different age groups?

- Where and how do we usually talk about sex?

- What are socially acceptable ways to talk about sexual intercourse? For example in English people say "sleeping with..." when they mean "having sexual intercourse with...." Point out that the problem with this euphemism is that it may mislead or confuse — because it is possible to sleep with someone without having sex and possible to have sex without sleeping with someone!

- What does "sexual health" mean to you?

GROUP DISCUSSION EXERCISE (CONTINUED): TALKING ABOUT SEXUALITY AND SEXUAL HEALTH

After five minutes ask the groups for their suggestions about the meaning of sexual health and write them up on a large sheet of paper. Then show a transparency or large sheet with the WHO definition of sexual health: "the integration of the physical, emotional, intellectual, and social aspects of sexual being, in ways that are enriching and that enhance personality, communication, and love."

Explain that if we want to promote sexual health we need to understand sex, sexuality, sexually transmitted infections, and the social factors that influence sexual behavior.

If education about safer sex is to be effective it has to be based on what people really do rather than on what society says people should do. "Sexuality" is about more than sexual practices and includes the relationships in which they occur.

Next ask the groups to discuss:

• What are some of the reasons why men have sex?

• What are some of the reasons why women have sex?

After five minutes put all the reasons up on paper. Point out that there is a spectrum of what is sometimes called "transactional sex." Someone may exchange sex for love, protection, financial security, luxuries, essentials such as food or clothing, or money — and this may be a single incident or a long relationship. This understanding can help to change judgmental attitudes toward sex workers.

Then ask them to discuss:

• How do children and young people learn about sex?

• How did you learn about sex yourself? Did you learn about self-confidence, respect, and relationships as well as the facts about sex?

• What sexual practices are common and acceptable for men, for women?

• How common is homosexuality? Do homosexual men tend to live with other men or do they marry but continue to have sex with other men? What are attitudes toward male and female homosexuality?

• What happens to men and women who break society's "rules" for acceptable sexual behavior?

After the discussion ask the participants to discuss for a moment how they felt about talking freely about sexual matters. Is it easier to talk about other people's sexual behavior than your own?

The book *Where Women Have No Doctor* has an excellent chapter on sexual health, which provides useful material for discussion. See A. August Burns et al., *Where Women Have No Doctor: A Health Guide for Women* (New York: Macmillan, 1997).

Checking knowledge—
basic facts about HIV

To prevent the spread of HIV we need to have a good understanding of the way that the virus behaves, how it spreads, and the way that it affects the body.

"Basic Facts" (chapter 2) provides information about the virus, stages of infection, definition of AIDS, tests for HIV, transmission routes, surveillance, and treatment. More detailed information is included elsewhere in the manual. For example, "Basic Facts" describes the different tests for HIV, but testing strategies are described in appendix B (page 199). In addition, the chapter explains how the virus passes from an infected mother, but the interventions to prevent parent-to-child transmission are described in chapter 11.

Depending on the level of knowledge of the staff you might want to go through "Basic Facts," have a question-and-answer session, or simply distribute the section as a handout. Scientists' understanding of HIV is increasing all the time. It is important to stay up to date with these advances in knowledge. Some useful newsletters are mentioned under "Additional resources" and the websites and mailing lists are a good source of information if you have access to the Internet.

2

Basic Facts about HIV Infection

Acquired Immune Deficiency Syndrome (AIDS) is a new and fatal disease caused by a virus called the Human Immunodeficiency Virus, or HIV. Since the early 1980s it has spread rapidly and is having a serious impact on the social and economic structure of many countries. In some areas AIDS has become a major threat to child survival. Productive young adults are becoming ill and dying, which leaves children and the elderly without support.

THE VIRUS

AIDS was first described in the United States in 1981, but the virus that causes the immune deficiency was not discovered until 1983. HIV infects and damages or destroys the white blood cells of the body that make up the immune system.

Like other viruses, HIV is able to reproduce only inside the cells of the infected person. Viruses contain genetic instructions (the genome), but they lack the machinery to make new viruses. In most groups of viruses the genome remains separate from the host cell genome, and the body is able to eliminate the infection. However, the genome of HIV integrates with the genome of the host cell. When the infected host cells multiply each new cell contains the HIV genome. In this way, HIV remains permanently in the infected person. When infected cells are stimulated they produce new viruses.

There are two viruses that cause immune deficiency: HIV-1 and HIV-2. In this manual we use HIV to refer to the more common virus, HIV-1. HIV-2 is transmitted in the same ways as HIV-1, but it is less infectious and infected people remain well longer. HIV-2 was first identified in West Africa, where it remains common,

but it has also since been identified in many parts of the world, including Asia.

The virus is sensitive to heat and is killed at 56°C. It is able to survive outside the body only for a brief period, which depends on the temperature and fluid around the virus.

STAGES OF INFECTION

Seroconversion

During the first few weeks after exposure to the virus, HIV multiplies rapidly. Next, usually within three months, the person starts to produce antibodies to HIV. This process is called seroconversion. Antibodies are formed to several parts of the virus. However, most of these antibodies are not neutralizing antibodies; they cannot overcome the infection. The virus mutates frequently, especially the gene for the virus envelope (or coat) that is the part of the virus that the host's immune system recognizes first. This makes it difficult for the antibodies to recognize and destroy the virus.

Many people experience an acute illness at the time of seroconversion, with fever and enlarged lymph glands. Some have neurological symptoms. The illness lasts about fourteen days, and may be mistaken for infectious mononucleosis (glandular fever) or flu.

Latency

After this, most people infected with HIV have no symptoms for months or years. During this "latency" period the virus is reproducing slowly and there are low levels of virus in the blood. The HIV antibody test is positive. Later, the number of white cells decreases, the amount of virus in the blood increases, and infected people develop clinical disease. They may suffer a wide range of symptoms including loss

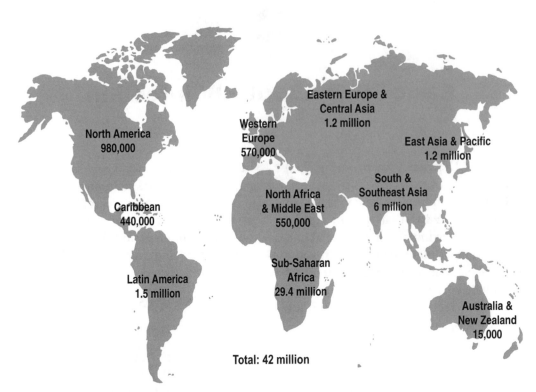

North America
980,000

Eastern Europe &
Central Asia
1.2 million

Western
Europe
570,000

East Asia & Pacific
1.2 million

Caribbean
440,000

North Africa
& Middle East
550,000

South &
Southeast Asia
6 million

Latin America
1.5 million

Sub-Saharan
Africa
29.4 million

Australia &
New Zealand
15,000

Total: 42 million

ADULTS AND CHILDREN ESTIMATED TO BE LIVING WITH HIV/AIDS AS OF THE END OF 2001. Source: UNAIDS, 2002

of weight, tiredness, fever, cough, and diarrhea. The latency period is long and variable, and may range from four months to more than ten years. A period of three years without symptoms is typical.

AIDS

Acquired Immune Deficiency Syndrome, or AIDS, is what we call the final stage of HIV infection when the immune system is very weak. Microorganisms are then able to take the opportunity to infect the person so these infections are called "opportunistic." The weak immune system may also allow cancers to develop. Tuberculosis, Pneumocystis carinii pneumonia, fungal infections, and cryptococcal meningitis are common opportunistic infections in AIDS patients. Kaposi's sarcoma, lymphoma, and cervical carcinoma are common cancers. Neurological disease, due to direct infection of brain cells by the virus, may occur early or late in the course of HIV infection. HIV-infected women may also

suffer from severe vaginal herpes, candidiasis (thrush), and pelvic inflammatory disease. The spread of tuberculosis is increased in the crowded conditions in which refugees and IDPs often live.

After infection with HIV about one-third of those infected will develop AIDS within five years; and about two-thirds will develop AIDS within twelve years. A small number of HIV-infected people have not developed symptoms or immune deficiency even after many years. Shorter times between HIV infection and the first signs of illness, and shorter survival times with AIDS, have been reported in poor countries in comparison with richer countries. Differential access to new combination antiviral therapies and to antibiotics that prevent and treat opportunistic infections are increasing these differences.

Where laboratory resources are available doctors can measure the white cell count and the viral load to monitor the progress of the disease.

⚕ DISCUSSION POINT ⚕

There is strong evidence that HIV is the cause of AIDS. However, some people have suggested that it is not HIV that causes AIDS but poverty and abuse of drugs. HIV causes immune deficiency so people with AIDS may exhibit different patterns of illness because they have different opportunistic infections. This makes it easy for people to believe that AIDS is not a new and distinct disease. The way this virus behaves is not familiar to most people. But there are other viruses like HIV, that have a long incubation period before they cause illness, and that set up a permanent infection, such as hepatitis B or herpes simplex.

In fact, of course, there are many studies from all parts of the world that prove that people with AIDS test positive for HIV antibodies and for the virus itself. The virus has been isolated from the blood and tissues of people with HIV. We can see photographs of HIV taken through a very powerful microscope. The U.S. Centers for Disease Control and Prevention have produced a paper providing the evidence to counter some of the many myths that people believe about HIV, available at *www.niaid.nih.gov*.

Why do you think people believe these myths? What are the effects when policy makers hold and promote these false beliefs?

CASE DEFINITION OF AIDS

The U.S. Centers for Disease Control and Prevention (CDC) definition of AIDS is complicated and has changed several times. It depends on the diagnosis of at least one of a list of diseases that indicate immune deficiency and includes laboratory evidence of HIV infection and a low T4 white cell count.

Where there are no facilities for the diagnosis of indicator diseases or the detection of HIV antibodies, the World Health Organization clinical definition may be used (see p. 22). However, this definition is not very accurate in diagnosing persons with HIV infection because it includes symptoms and signs that may be common in uninfected individuals in developing countries, such as chronic cough, weight loss, and recurrent fever. Some countries use their own modification of the clinical definition.

PROGNOSIS

Where antiviral treatment and prophylaxis for opportunistic infections are not available, people usually die within a year of diagnosis of AIDS. Where intensive monitoring and treatment are available, people with AIDS may live for many years. The main causes of death among patients with AIDS in developing countries are chronic diarrhea, chest infection, tuberculosis, cryptococcal meningitis, and disseminated Kaposi's sarcoma.

TESTS FOR HIV INFECTION

The first blood test for HIV was developed in 1985. It was a test for the antibodies to HIV, not for the virus itself. Therefore in the early stage of infection, before antibodies have been produced, it is possible for infected persons to test negative. Infected people usually test positive for HIV antibodies within one month after infection. However, in a small number of people this may take three months or more (the "window period"). When people become very ill with AIDS they may stop making antibodies to the virus so the antibody test may be negative. However, they are still able to transmit the virus to other people.

WHO GUIDELINES FOR CLINICAL DIAGNOSIS OF AIDS IN ADULTS

Major signs	• Weight loss of over 10 percent of body weight • Fever for longer than one month • Diarrhea for longer than one month
Minor signs	• Persistent cough for more than one month • General itchy skin rash • Recurring shingles (herpes zoster) • Thrush in the mouth and throat • Long-lasting, spreading, and severe cold sores (herpes simplex) • Long-lasting and symmetrical swelling of the lymph glands (general lymphadenopathy) • Loss of memory • Loss of intellectual capacity • Peripheral nerve damage
At least two major and at least one minor sign in an adult, in the absence of any other clear explanation for the signs (such as cancer or malnutrition), defines AIDS.	

Purposes of HIV antibody testing

- diagnosis, when a patient has signs and symptoms suggestive of HIV;

- as part of voluntary counseling and testing services, when individuals want to know their HIV status;

- prenatal screening, when interventions are available to reduce the risk of mother-to-child transmission;

- screening of donated blood for transfusion;

- surveillance, to provide data about the extent of spread of the epidemic; and

- research.

The different types of HIV tests are described in chapter 8.

TRANSMISSION OF HIV

HIV spreads in three ways: (1) through sexual intercourse, (2) through blood, and (3) from mother to child.

The virus is not transmitted by coughing or sneezing, shaking hands, sharing a cup or plate, hugging or kissing, insect bites, spitting, or by living or working with someone who has HIV infection or AIDS.

People are more infectious shortly after they become infected and again when they later develop the signs of damage to their immune system. This is because there is a greater viral load, or concentration of virus in the bloodstream and other bodily fluids, at these times.

The pattern of transmission depends on behavior patterns and varies from place to place and in different groups within a population.

Transmission through sex

Vaginal sexual intercourse is the most common route of transmission of HIV. Anal sex (whether male-male, or male-female) carries a higher risk of transmission than vaginal sex.

Sexually transmitted infections (STIs), especially those that cause genital sores or ulcers, increase the risk of getting and of passing on HIV for both men and women. Chlamydia and gonorrhea, which cause a discharge, are more common than ulcerative STIs such as syphilis or chancroid. They may cause no symptoms and so remain untreated for long periods. For these reasons they may be relatively more important than ulcerative STIs in adding to the risk of transmission. Other infections of the reproductive tract that are not necessarily sexually transmitted, including thrush (candidiasis) and bacterial infections (bacterial vaginosis) also increase vulnerability to HIV. These are common and easily treatable conditions. The probability of infection from a single act of vaginal intercourse when both partners have healthy genitals is very small — about one in one thousand. So preventing STIs and providing effective treatment are important strategies to prevent the spread of HIV.

Young women are especially vulnerable to HIV. HIV is more likely to spread when sexual activity is rough or repeated frequently. Anything that increases the risk of damage to the skin of the vagina such as the practice of using herbs and other substances to dry and heat the vagina, or use of sex "toys," is likely to increase the risk of transmission. There is evidence that uncircumcised men are at greater risk of becoming infected with HIV than circumcised men. Both male and female condoms reduce the risk of transmission through sexual intercourse (see page 91).

Transmission through blood

Blood transfusion

A transfusion of blood from a donor infected with HIV will infect the patient who receives it. Whole blood, red blood cells, platelets, and plasma may contain HIV. HIV can also be transmitted from one person to another through transplantation of any organ or tissue. Routine testing of all blood for transfusion greatly reduces the chances of transmitting HIV this way, but there always remains a small risk because of the "window period" (see page 21). Strict criteria for blood transfusion can reduce the frequency of transfusions greatly without increase in deaths. The viruses hepatitis B and C can also spread through blood transfusions.

Needle-stick injury

Needle-stick accidents and blood splashes to the mouth or eyes in the health care setting may lead to the infection of health care workers. The risk is very low and can be reduced further by strict attention to universal infection control precautions (see page 170).

Injecting drug use

Injecting drug use is becoming increasingly common in many countries, especially in Asia and Eastern Europe. HIV, and hepatitis B and C, spread very easily between people who inject drugs together and share needles, syringes, and other injecting equipment. Blood drawn back into the syringe can pass directly into the bloodstream of the next person to use the syringe, so infection is almost certain. HIV may then spread from infected drug users to others in the population through sexual intercourse.

Transmission from mother to child

HIV can pass from an infected woman to her baby during pregnancy, at the time of delivery, or afterward through breast-feeding. Not all babies born to a mother with HIV become infected with HIV. The risk of infection for babies varies greatly between the different groups studied. When there is no breast-feeding the percentage that become infected is between 15 and 30. In breast-feeding populations the percentage of babies that become infected is between 30 and 45. The virus is most likely to pass to the baby during labor or in the first few weeks of breast-feeding, although a small proportion become infected earlier in the pregnancy.

HIV antibodies from the mother cross the placenta to the baby so the HIV antibody test is positive at birth whether the baby is infected or not. These maternal antibodies stay in the baby for as long as eighteen months, although most babies lose maternal HIV antibodies by nine months of age.

The virus is more likely to pass to the baby if the woman is newly infected. This is because the level of HIV in the blood is very high a few weeks after infection with the virus. After this the body starts to fight the virus and the level in the blood becomes very low. It usually stays low for several years. The risk of transmission to the baby is also high when the mother develops symptoms and signs of AIDS and the amount of HIV in the blood rises again.

The risk also depends on the health of the woman: it is higher when she has other infections, especially infection of the placenta and amniotic fluid, and STIs, and when there are poor maternal weight gain and micronutrient deficiencies.

The risk is increased by invasive procedures such as amniocentesis and artificial rupture of membranes. It is possible, but not yet proved, that episiotomy and certain practices of traditional midwives, such as firm abdominal massage, may increase the risk. Caesarean section performed before labor begins reduces the risk of transmitting HIV to the baby.

The baby of an HIV-infected woman may remain uninfected during pregnancy and delivery but become infected through breast-feeding. Other babies become infected when their mothers become infected after the birth during the period of lactation. The only randomized controlled trial of breast-feeding versus formula was conducted in Kenya and found an increased risk of transmission in breast-fed babies of 16 percent.

The risk is higher when a woman becomes infected with HIV during the period of lactation, because of the post-infection rise in viral load. Most breast milk HIV transmission occurs early during breast-feeding, although some risk continues throughout the period of breast-feeding. Most babies born to HIV-infected mothers who are breast fed do not become infected with HIV and may benefit from the general and HIV-specific antibodies in breast milk.

The risk of infection through breast-feeding is increased by inflammation of the breast, such as mastitis or an abscess. There is evidence that exclusive breast-feeding, when the baby receives nothing but breast milk, may be safer than mixed feeding (breast milk and other fluids).

There is a range of strategies to reduce the number of babies with HIV. These are described in chapter 11.

Our knowledge about the factors that influence the risk of transmission of HIV is changing rapidly. It is important to keep up to date with changes through newsletters, journal articles, and, if you are able to access it, the Internet.

EPIDEMIOLOGY AND SURVEILLANCE

UNAIDS/WHO uses the following classification to describe the HIV epidemic:

- a "generalized" epidemic is one where HIV prevalence has reached at least 1 percent among the general population;

- a "concentrated" epidemic is one where HIV prevalence has exceeded 5 percent among certain subpopulations; and

- a "low prevalence" epidemic is one in which infection remains below 5 percent in any given subpopulation.

Most sub-Saharan African countries suffer generalized epidemics. In many countries of the former Soviet Union and Eastern Europe there are rapidly increasing epidemics concentrated among people who inject drugs. Many countries in Southeast Asia currently have "low prevalence" epidemics. However, this may change rapidly, and there is evidence that incidence of HIV is rising rapidly in certain population groups such as sex workers and their clients, those who inject drugs, and men who have sex with men. Several southern and central states of India have generalized epidemics.

Surveillance means collecting data on HIV infection rates in a systematic way so that it is possible to follow trends in the prevalence of HIV infection in different groups within a population. Surveillance data is valuable for deciding which interventions and groups to prioritize.

The pattern of HIV transmission in populations that have been forced to migrate is likely to differ from that in stable settings. Sentinel surveillance is likely to be difficult in most humanitarian settings because it relies on a functioning and accessible health care system and some stability in composition of the groups that are sampled over time. Suggestions for gaining information about the extent of spread of HIV in forced migrant populations are described in part 2.

TREATMENT FOR HIV INFECTION

At present, there is no cure for AIDS. However, there are treatments for the relief of symptoms, treatments for opportunistic infections, and an increasing range of antiretroviral drugs that attack HIV itself.

Unfortunately the countries that have the largest numbers of people infected with HIV are unable to afford the high cost of the new antiretroviral drug combinations; many cannot afford to provide treatment for opportunistic infections; and many people affected by HIV are unable even to afford medicines to relieve symptoms.

Good nursing care can do much to relieve the symptoms of HIV-related disease such as fever, sweating, itching, diarrhea, pain, headache, and cough. Local homemade remedies and traditional healers can be very helpful. Paracetamol, aspirin, oral rehydration solution, gentian violet, and antiseptic cream are useful, and morphine, if it is available, helps to relieve pain in dying patients at low cost (see page 179). Nutrition and food preparation advice is also important.

Treatment for opportunistic infections such as tuberculosis, diarrhea, fungal infections, and *Pneumocystis carinii* pneumonia can extend and improve the life of people living with HIV and their family. Effective low-cost generic drugs for opportunistic infections should be on "essential drugs lists" and available to those who need them. It is important to treat tuberculosis both for the individual and the community. Thrush (candidiasis), toxoplasmosis, and pneumonia can be treated at low cost, which may enable a person with HIV to live for several more years.

A person with HIV can take isoniazid to prevent tuberculosis and co-trimoxazole to prevent other bacterial infections. These are called prophylactic medicines.

Antiretroviral drugs kill HIV and so reduce the level of virus in the blood. A combination of these drugs needs to be taken for life, and they often have side effects. People living with HIV/AIDS (PLWH/A) who are able to access these drugs can remain well for many years, although the virus remains in the body. However, despite recent price reductions these drugs remain out of reach for most PLWH/A (see page 182).

TEN COMMONLY ASKED QUESTIONS

Answering these questions often provides an opportunity to explore attitudes and to correct common misunderstandings.

1. Where did HIV come from?

We are still not certain about the origin of HIV. It is likely that HIV evolved from similar viruses, called simian immunodeficiency viruses (SIVs), found to infect monkeys. It is possible that an SIV transferred to humans in central Africa as a result of hunting and handling of chimpanzee meat. The first documented case of HIV-1 infection occurred in 1959 in a man living in what is now the Democratic Republic of Congo.

The suggestion that humans may have been infected with SIV through vaccination with a contaminated oral polio vaccine has been discounted. There is no scientific evidence that HIV came from space or from a germ warfare laboratory.

2. Why didn't public health doctors isolate people with HIV from the beginning to prevent it spreading, as they do for other diseases?

By the time that the virus that causes AIDS was identified there were already many people infected with HIV. Most people with HIV do not know that they are infected. If those known to be infected were isolated, the rest of the population might feel that they are not at risk and that there would be no need to change high-risk behavior or to protect themselves against infection. People would not come forward for testing if they knew that they would be isolated. Even if it were possible to screen everyone in the population at once, there would still be some infected people who test negative because of the window period. People infected with HIV usually remain well for many years. Isolating people for life is a violation of their human rights.

3. Mosquitoes spread malaria and dengue fever. How do we know that they don't spread HIV?

This subject has been carefully researched. There are several reasons why we can be sure that HIV does not spread through mosquito bites:

- Studies show that, even in places where there are lots of mosquitoes and HIV infection is common, elderly people and children often get bitten by mosquitoes but do not become infected with HIV.

- When an insect bites a person, it does not inject any blood, only saliva.

- Researchers have studied mosquitoes in the laboratory, allowing them to suck up HIV-infected blood and then killing and examining them. They find that HIV cannot survive or reproduce inside the mosquito's stomach (unlike the malaria parasite). So the mosquito cannot transmit HIV to the next person it bites.

- Mosquitoes do not bite one person straight after another — they rest after they have sucked blood from one person.

4. When will we have a vaccine for HIV? Why is it taking researchers so long?

Although research laboratories around the world are trying to develop vaccines against HIV, a safe, reliable vaccine is unlikely to become available for many years. Researchers are trying to develop two types of vaccine: one to prevent infection with HIV and the other to prevent progression to AIDS once someone is already infected with the virus.

Vaccines usually work by making the body produce antibodies that attack the virus or bacteria. The envelope pattern of HIV mutates (changes) frequently. Antibodies are unable to recognize the virus, so they cannot attack it.

Once a vaccine is developed there are many problems to overcome, including testing of the vaccine and effective distribution. These involve many complex ethical, legal, and sociopolitical issues. The International AIDS Vaccine Initiative is working to evaluate trial vaccines and to provide up-to-date information on the progress of vaccine development (website: *www.iavi.org*).

5. How is it possible that there are couples where the husband is infected and the wife is not, or where the wife is infected and the husband is not?

There are many cases of couples where one has the virus and the other has not, even though they have had sex many times. The risk of transmission through sex is very low when there are no STIs and when sexual practices do not damage the skin of the genital organs. Some people have a lower risk than others of becoming infected after being exposed to HIV. This may be related to the strain of the virus, the level of the person's immune system, and genetic factors that are not yet well understood. When a couple is tested and one is found to be infected with HIV, it is important to recommend condom use during sex and to explain that although the partner has not yet become infected this does not mean that it could not happen.

6. Is it true that an infected man is more likely to pass on HIV than an infected woman?

Studies from Europe suggested that HIV passes from an infected man to a woman during sex more easily than it passes from an infected woman to a man. However, a large study from Uganda found the opposite.[1]

7. How can it be that some babies born to HIV-infected women are not infected with HIV?

Many people assume that all babies born to a mother infected with HIV will also be infected with HIV because they think that the baby shares the same blood supply as the mother in the womb. In fact the blood circulation of the growing baby and of the mother are separated in the placenta by a layer of cells. Oxygen, nutrients, antibodies, and some medicines can pass across this cell barrier, but usually HIV does not. If the placenta is inflamed or damaged

1. R. H. Gray et al. and the Rakai Project Team, "Probability of HIV-1 Transmission per Coital Act in Monogamous, Heterosexual, HIV-1–Discordant Couples in Rakai, Uganda," *Lancet* 357 (2001): 1149–53, April 14, 2001, held at HSL.

it is easier for the virus to cross the cell barrier and the risk that the baby will be infected increases. There is often some mixing of the baby's and mother's blood during labor, and exposure of the baby to the mother's blood during delivery, so this is the time when HIV transmission is most likely to occur. But most babies of HIV-positive women do not become infected with HIV.

Factors that increase the risk of transmission of HIV from mother to baby are described in "Basic Facts" (see page 23).

8. Once a person has tested positive for HIV, can that person become negative again—even without treatment?

HIV, unlike most viruses, sets up a permanent infection in the body. The genetic material of the virus merges with the genetic material of the host cells. A positive test for HIV means that the person has antibodies to HIV. It is possible, although rare, to have a false positive result. If this happens another test in the future might test negative.

But if a person is infected, then the HIV test will usually stay positive. Sometimes the immune system can be so damaged by HIV that the person stops making antibodies to HIV and the test may become negative, even though the person is still infected and able to infect others.

A few people infected with HIV continue to have a positive antibody test, but remain well for much longer than the average. It may be that some people are able to keep HIV at such low levels in their body that they never develop signs and symptoms of HIV-related immune deficiency.

9. How reliable is the HIV antibody test? I heard that it could be positive if you've had measles.

The first antibody tests used mashed-up HIV. They cross-reacted with many other antibodies that resulted in a high rate of false positives. People who had had multiple infections in the past were more likely to test positive, so there were more false positive results in African than in European populations. Newer tests use genetically engineered components of HIV and have fewer false positives.

The first objective of developing a test for HIV was to screen blood for transfusions. The cut-off point for the test was therefore designed to decrease the chance that an infected sample would falsely test negative, that is, the test needed to be very sensitive. Tests that are very sensitive tend to be less specific and result in higher rates of false positives. Modern antibody tests are very sensitive and very specific. Most ELISA tests have a sensitivity between 99 and 100 percent and a specificity between 98 and 100 percent. The simple rapid tests are as sensitive, but some are a little less specific.

10. Why won't a complete transfusion of blood, like an exchange transfusion for a jaundiced baby, cure someone with HIV?

HIV infects white cells in the blood, but the virus does not stay only in the blood. The virus spreads to other parts of the immune system, including the lymph nodes, the spleen, and the liver. The virus can also infect cells in the brain and in the intestine. So even if you could completely change the blood in the body, this would not cure the person, and HIV in the person's body would soon enter the bloodstream again.

ADDITIONAL RESOURCES

AEGIS (AIDS Education Global Information System). *www.aegis.com.*

CDC, Division of HIV/AIDS Prevention (DHAP). *www.cdc.gov.*

UNAIDS. "HIV/AIDS: The Global Epidemic." Geneva. Annual updates. Summarizes the status and trends of the epidemic. Includes global and regional estimates and selected examples on the epidemic in specific countries and regions. *www.unaids.org.*

UNAIDS. "Trends in HIV Incidence and Prevalence: Natural Course of the Epidemic or Results of Behavioral Change?" UNAIDS in collaboration with Wellcome Trust Centre for the Epidemiology of Infectious Disease. UNAIDS, Geneva. June 1999. Available at *www.aegis.com/files/unaids/WAD1999_trends_report.pdf.*

WHO. WHO fact sheets on HIV/AIDS for nurses and midwives. *www.who.int.*

WHO. "Sexually Transmitted Infections." *www.who.int.* This WHO Communicable Disease Surveillance and Response site includes information on HIV/AIDS and sexually transmitted infections as well as links to many other AIDS-related sites.

3

Thinking about the Communities You Work With

UNDERSTANDING VULNERABILITY AND RESILIENCE

HIV spreads through the behaviors of individuals, but these behaviors are influenced by the social and cultural context. To plan for prevention and care we need to understand this context and how the community is affected by displacement due to armed conflict. The impact of displacement may lead to behaviors that increase vulnerability to HIV and affects the way that the community responds to the epidemic.

NGO staff work in a wide range of contexts. The effects of displacement will depend on the beneficiary population's culture, their current situation and composition, experiences during the conflict, length of time since they were displaced, the status of the conflict that led to their displacement, and their prospects for returning home. In resettled communities the morale and outlook of the population will depend on whether they feel defeated or victorious.

Ask the team to think about the consequences of displacement for the people that they work with (including the host population). Make a list of these down the left-hand side of a large sheet of paper. Then ask what effects these may have on refugees, IDPs, and other conflict-affected populations. Write these characteristics to the right of the list of consequences. "Understanding Vulnerability to HIV" on page 30 shows the outcome of one team of staff's discussion.

In such environments behaviors that facilitate the spread of HIV and STIs are likely to be common. Social life is disrupted, along with the usual patterns of sexual behavior. There is likely to be a lack of opportunities for social activities that enable men and women to meet in culturally acceptable ways. There may be an increase in casual sex, sex in exchange for food, goods, or protection, coerced sex, commercial sex, and high rates of sexual assault and rape. Local or international military and the host population may be interacting sexually with refugees/IDPs and may have higher rates of sexually transmitted infections and HIV. Blood may be transfused without screening, and access to health care is limited. There may be excessive use of drugs and alcohol, and antisocial behavior such as stealing, vandalism, and violence.

The roles and responsibilities of men and women, and the relationships between them, are often dramatically altered when populations are displaced as a result of conflict. Nevertheless both men and women continue to be influenced by the gender roles and relations that prevailed in their own communities. It is important to think about the differences in impact of displacement for men and for women.

Women's reproductive health and vulnerability to STIs and HIV are greatly affected by men, whose behavior is influenced by their experiences during and after armed conflict. Men may be traumatized by torture or rape, feel guilty because they failed to protect their family, or perhaps committed atrocities themselves. They may be depressed, lonely, and bored. Men generally have few emotional outlets and lose their role in refugee/IDP camps, while women's work of caring for children, cleaning, cooking, and collecting fuel continues. One man in a camp in Tanzania said, "UNHCR is now my wife's husband."

Similarly the impact will be different for different age groups. Encourage the group to talk

UNDERSTANDING VULNERABILITY TO HIV

Consequences of displacement due to armed conflict	*Characteristics*

Multiple losses
  – deaths of family/friends
  – home
  – land
  – job/school
	sadness
	bereavement
	depression

Uncertain future	fatalism desire to go home short-term view
Loss of legal status; rights; autonomy	apathy fear
Dependence on camp routines and regulations	insecurity anxiety loneliness

Breakdown of family and social structures
  – increase in proportions of single men,
    and women-headed households
	suspicion
	lack of trust
	lack of respect

Impoverishment	hunger
Loss of services	poor health stress

Suffered traumatic events:
  – captivity
  – rape
  – torture
  – witnessed deaths
  – committed atrocities
	numbness
	guilt

Lack of meaningful activity	boredom aggression frustration
New influences	risk-taking

about differences between how children, young people, adults, and the elderly experience the changes forced on them by displacement.

Consider whether there are any strengths or positive outcomes from the community's experiences. These might include:

- feelings of belonging and solidarity within the group—shared sense of identity;

- awareness of resilience and ability to endure;

- strong women—women's role maintained;

- increased opportunities for women to be independent;

- time to be involved with communication and behavior change activities, and with care for those infected and affected.

Finally ask the team to think about the attitudes and behavior of the host population in relation to the refugees and IDPs. Are they sympathetic and supportive, or resentful of the resources and services provided for the refugees/IDPs?

Although it is important to have an understanding of the culture and characteristics of the community, we should be careful not to stereotype people. Ask the staff to think about how well they fit within their own culture. Few people think of themselves as typical.

Once you have built up a picture of the impact of displacement on the community, invite the staff to get into smaller groups. Ask them to discuss the implications of these characteristics for the community's vulnerability to HIV and for their capacity to respond.

IMPACT OF THE EPIDEMIC

The impacts of the epidemic depend on the prevalence and pattern of HIV infection among the refugees/IDPs and in the host population.

For political reasons it is often difficult to obtain information about rates of HIV among refugees/IDPs. If information exists it may be difficult to access. Surveillance studies may not have been carried out for logistical reasons, or out of fear that the host government or resettlement countries might not accept refugees/IDPs if they fear that they may have HIV.

Some assessment of the likely prevalence of HIV may be made by considering:

- the rate in the population that the refugees/IDPs have come from,

- the rate, if known, in the host population,

- other markers of risk such as high rates of sexually transmitted infections, sexual violence, or injecting drug use.

Ask the staff to think about likely impacts in the setting in which you work. These might include:

- increased burden of illness,

- decreased ability to work — whether subsistence farming or paid jobs,

- possibility of spread of tuberculosis if many people have HIV-related immune deficiency,

- increased need for health care services and medicines,

- strain on already stretched health care workers and counselors,

- increased burden on women caring for sick relatives or children,

- increased numbers of orphans needing care,

- increased vulnerability of young people left without parents,

- emotional and mental health problems caused by discrimination and stigma,

- fear of rejection by host country, home country, or resettlement country.

4

What Role Might NGOs Play in the Response to HIV?

Take some time to discuss what role your team might play in response to the needs for HIV prevention and care. This will vary greatly from one setting to another and will depend on:

- the prevalence of HIV in the population from which the refugees/IDPs have come;

- the prevalence of HIV in the host population;

- the level of risk factors;

- the type of setting: refugee/IDP camp; refugee-impacted area; or resettlement area;

- the degree of stability and security;

- whether the refugees'/IDPs' current circumstances are anticipated to be short- or long-term;

- the types of programs that your organization is already implementing;

- existing responses that may have been initiated by the host government, UN agencies, international NGOs, local NGOs, and the community.

What aspects of your work already contribute to reducing vulnerability to HIV?

Examples might include:

- social activities that promote equality and respect, provide some relief from stress and anxiety, and enable men and women to meet in culturally acceptable ways;

- efforts to protect women from rape and coerced sex;

- sports activities for young people that give them confidence and hope for the future;

- prenatal, delivery, and postnatal care that improves the health of pregnant women,

minimizes interventions at delivery, and increases the likelihood of optimal exclusive breast-feeding — all measures that will reduce the risk of mother-to-child transmission of HIV (see chapter 11).

Often an increased awareness that their work contributes to HIV prevention and care raises the morale and commitment of staff.

How might HIV prevention and care be incorporated into existing programs?

There may be ways to build in responses immediately without the need for additional resources:

- in a program for young people a poster competition could have the theme "reducing stigma associated with HIV infection";

- inviting a panel of community leaders to be the judges may also engage them in the issue;

- a women's literacy program might use material with HIV-related topics; the AIDS Action newsletters (see appendix E, page 216) are a useful source of material to stimulate discussions;

- community health workers who undertake home visits could be trained to provide one-to-one education about HIV and STIs and to distribute condoms;

- during supervisory visits to clinics staff can ensure that appropriate measures are in place to prevent transmission of HIV in the health care setting, and that simple opportunities to contribute to HIV prevention and care are not being missed.

Encourage the team to think of ideas for your setting.

What HIV-related issues should NGOs address because of particular designated responsibilities?

For example, if your NGO has responsibility for health care services, the organization also has a responsibility to ensure that measures are in place to minimize the risk of transmission in health care settings and to provide nondiscriminatory counseling, care, and support to people infected and affected by HIV.

Which organization in your setting is responsible for coordinating the implementation of MISP?

The components of the evidence-based Minimum Initial Service Package for reproductive health form a minimum requirement of actions in the emergency phase (see page 35). In your setting, which organization is responsible for coordinating the implementation of MISP? To what extent has the package been implemented and monitored?

Next steps

In addition to strengthening what is already being done, the team may feel that there is a need for a greater or more comprehensive response to the threat of HIV. Coordination, collaboration, and communication are as important in relation to HIV interventions as to other interventions in humanitarian settings. Before new responses are implemented there will need to be an analysis of the situation with review of existing responses. This should include all those with an interest. The findings provide the basis for strategic planning.

HIV prevention and care efforts need to fit within the policy framework of the host government. It is important to become familiar with national AIDS control plans, policies, and programs.

In any setting consultation is important, but in refugee and IDP communities it assumes an even greater significance. HIV is a sensitive issue — a stigmatized condition surrounded by misconceptions. It is associated with illegal and stigmatized behaviors such as injecting drug use, sexual assault, and sex work. Gathering information about these issues can put people at risk and needs to be done cautiously, with full consultation and using participatory methods. But gathering information can be difficult in often-chaotic humanitarian settings, where there may be high mobility and security concerns. In particular confidentiality can be difficult to maintain, but it is essential.

There is a need to plan consultation carefully. There are inevitably delicate political tensions to take into account, and a range of stakeholders. These might include:

- officials of the host government,
- community leaders (of different factions),
- representatives of people living with HIV,
- military officials,
- religious leaders,
- representatives of UNHCR and other UN agencies, and
- other local or international humanitarian agencies and NGOs.

Consultation may be at several levels. For some stakeholders it may be appropriate to simply inform them of what is planned through a meeting. Others might be invited to comment on plans, while some will need the opportunity to participate fully in the cycle of gathering information, strategic planning, implementation, and evaluation.

Brainstorm with the team a list of people who need to be consulted. Go through the list deciding what level of consultation is appropriate for each stakeholder. Decide what will be the best approach and who will make contact. For example, you might invite people to an initial large open meeting to determine the level of interest and support, or organize a number of smaller consultations.

The next part describes how to undertake a situation analysis, response review, and strategic planning process.

Part 2

ENGAGING THE COMMUNITY

Part 2 deals with how to engage the local community. Different settings require different strategies. There will always be a need to gather information in a participatory way to inform local strategic planning, to consult closely with local stakeholders, and to engage community members in the response to the epidemic.

MINIMUM INITIAL SERVICES PACKAGE

Current humanitarian standards include a Minimum Initial Services Package (MISP) of reproductive health activities to be provided in emergencies.[1] These activities, designed to reduce reproductive health morbidity and mortality, should be put in place before any situation analysis in new refugee/IDP situations. MISP activities to reduce the transmission of HIV include:

- identifying an individual and organization responsible for ensuring that the MISP is implemented;

- ensuring a safe blood supply;

- implementing universal precautions for strict infection control;

- guaranteeing the availability of free condoms;

- addressing the prevention and management of sexual violence; and

- planning for comprehensive reproductive health services, including a site-specific HIV/AIDS situation analysis.

STRATEGIC PLANNING

In the post-emergency phase relevant organizations and a range of representatives from the refugee/IDP and host populations will need to plan additional STI and HIV prevention and care strategies. The type of setting and the degree of stability and security will determine which interventions will be feasible and appropriate.

In part 2 we consider how to plan a more comprehensive response to the threat of HIV. Strategic planning is based on a solid understanding of the local situation, risk factors, and existing responses. Analyzing the situation means identifying the most important routes of transmission of HIV, the influences on them, and the likely long-term impacts. It is complemented by a review of existing responses which identifies achievements and gaps.

Part 2 discusses process and methods for gathering information for the situation analysis and response review. It includes discussion of ethical issues, examples of topics that might be included, and ways to analyze and present the findings. We make some suggestions to guide the strategic planning process, including the planning for evaluation of interventions. UNAIDS has produced a four-module guide that can be helpful to the strategic planning process.[2]

The findings from the situation analysis and response review enable you to:

- decide how best to use existing resources,

- set priorities,

---

1. The SPHERE Project, Humanitarian Charter and Minimum Standards in Disaster Response, Geneva 2000.

2. *UNAIDS Guide to the Strategic Planning Process for a National Response to HIV/AIDS, www.unaids.org.*

- decide how best to reach different groups in the displaced and host populations,

- choose appropriate interventions and messages,

- identify obstacles to and opportunities for developing effective responses,

- decide how best to mobilize the capacity of the community and to obtain new resources, and

- plan how to monitor and evaluate activities and provide baseline data against which to measure progress.

Strategic planning should be realistic and includes considering the practical details of managing implementation of the strategies, such as who will do what, when, and how.

A good way to begin is to invite those you have identified as stakeholders (see "Next steps" in chapter 4, page 34) to a meeting to plan a situation analysis and response review.

The government of the country the refugees have come from and the host government may have developed national strategic plans. It is important to be aware of these plans to be able to take advantage of existing programs (for example, pre-tested education materials may be available that would be appropriate to use in the refugee/IDP setting), and to ensure that the strategic plan for the refugee/IDP community does not undermine or conflict with national policies and priorities. The strategic plan for the refugee/IDP community could be incorporated with the national plan as a special section for a priority group.

The process of bringing together key stakeholders for planning can be a powerful way to raise awareness and contribute to HIV prevention.

5

Gathering Information—
Analyzing the Situation

This chapter looks at the process of gathering relevant information for a situation analysis, the response review, and the presentation of the findings, in preparation for the strategic planning process itself, dealt with in chapter 6. We first consider the relevant topics of interest for the situation analysis and response review, and then the various methods for gathering information. We look at the process, including reviewing existing data and both quantitative and qualitative methods of gathering new data, and the ethical considerations that must be borne in mind during this process. We consider the response review, which looks at what is already being done; and then we consider how to present the findings. Chapter 5 ends with a summary guide to planning the entire process covered in the chapter.

TOPICS OF INTEREST

The selection or prioritizing of strategies and interventions for HIV prevention and care will depend on:

- the type of setting: refugee/IDP camp; refugee-impacted area; or resettlement area;

- the degree of stability and security;

- the prevalence of HIV in the population from which the refugees/IDPs have come;

- the prevalence of HIV in the host population;

- the composition of the refugee or displaced population;

- the level and pattern of risk factors;

- whether the refugees'/IDPs' current circumstances are anticipated to be short- or long-term;

- the types of social welfare, education, and health programs already being implemented;

- existing responses to HIV that may have been initiated by the host government, UN agencies, international NGOs, local NGOs, and the community.

The detailed planning of the strategies and interventions will depend on an understanding of:

- local decision-making structures and processes, networks, interest groups, and elites;

- gender roles and relations and the impact of displacement on these;

- the health status of the community;

- access to and use of health care and related services;

- patterns of sexual behavior and the influences on these;

- knowledge, attitudes, and practice in relation to STIs and HIV;

- management of blood safety and infection control;

- knowledge, attitudes, and practice in relation to injecting drug use;

- knowledge, beliefs, and practice in relation to pregnancy, childbirth, and infant feeding;

- care options for people with HIV-related illness;

- barriers to effective care and support for people living with HIV, including stigma;

- the laws that relate to HIV and other STIs.

During the situation analysis you need to gather together this information. Lists of questions to assist planning for the situation analysis are presented for each of these issues in appendix A (page 193). You may already have the answers to many of these questions, and some of the questions will not be relevant in your setting. An overview of the situation in relation to these issues may be sufficient for initial planning. A more extensive exploration of particular issues may be carried out later by the team that has responsibility for detailed planning and implementation of particular interventions.

METHODS FOR GATHERING INFORMATION

Methods that are useful for gathering information during a situation analysis and response review include:

- review of existing documents, databases, reports, books;

- focus group discussions;

- in-depth interviews with key informants;

- questionnaire surveys;

- observation;

- review of media — articles, editorials, letters;

- case studies — stories;

- participatory learning and action (PLA) techniques, such as mapping, matrix ranking, causal diagrams, and seasonal calendars.

We can classify different methods for gathering information into two main groups. Quantitative methods include questionnaire surveys, observation (with checklists), surveillance studies, and intervention studies. The results are usually in the form of numbers, percentages, tables, and graphs, e.g., morbidity and mortality data. Qualitative methods include focus group discussions, in-depth interviews, observation, and a variety of participatory exercises. The results or findings are usually in the form of words or pictures, often illustrated by quotes.

Sometimes researchers from different backgrounds suspect the validity of each other's methods. In reality both groups of methods are useful, and a combination of methods often provides the best understanding of an issue or problem. However, it is important to understand that the two groups of methods have different rules. Quantitative methods require random samples of adequate size and standardized questions so that the results can be extrapolated or generalized to the whole study population from which the sample is drawn. Qualitative results add a deeper understanding. These findings show the *range* of knowledge, attitudes, and practices or experiences. A sample is chosen deliberately, rather than randomly, to be representative of a group, such as "married women" or "clients of sex workers." The questions asked vary depending on the answers, so that we may learn things that we had not known to ask about.

It is important to collect information from a range of different sources to build up an accurate picture.

PROCESS

The *process* of gathering information provides an opportunity to establish links and trust with the community, raise awareness, and engage people in the response to the threat of HIV. However, the process can also undermine trust and cause harm if ethical implications are not carefully considered. This is especially important in humanitarian settings when there is often a high level of suspicion and fear, and when the topics of interest are sensitive.

Both qualitative and quantitative methods can be undertaken in a participatory way. When communities are closely involved with the gathering of information this will increase their understanding of how the research will benefit them. They will then be more likely to support it and ultimately use the findings. For example, local officials who train young people to be peer facilitators and then assist them in analyzing the data are likely to be convinced by the findings and motivated to make use of them in their planning. People also tend to speak more freely to their peers. Thus young people are more likely to give honest information to peer researchers than to older people. Finally, co-researchers from the community will be able to find creative ways to overcome obstacles that arise.

If there are people living with HIV who are willing to disclose their status publicly, they can play an important role in the situation analysis, planning, and implementation of activities.

"Outsiders" to the community can also play a useful role in the situation analysis if they are respectful and do not take control. They will have a different perspective and may suggest additional questions, notice different things, and be able to share lessons learned in other settings.

People who practice high-risk behaviors, such as having sex with sex workers or injecting drugs, and those who are vulnerable, such as young people, can be difficult groups to reach. Simply taking a nonjudgmental interest and trying to meet some of their needs can have a remarkable effect. Including them in the information-gathering process can help to produce reliable information and increase cooperation. It is important to take opportunities to collect information when they arise.

For example, if sex workers have gathered for any reason, such as a festival, you might take the opportunity to start a discussion, with their permission, about their knowledge and beliefs. This approach is likely to be more effective than making an appointment for a discussion at a particular date and time.

It is a good idea for each member of the team to carry a notebook during the period of the situation analysis to capture ideas, insights, and observations.

When deciding what topics to include and what questions to ask, it is important to think about how the information will be used. Beware of gathering too much information. It takes a long time to collect and analyze data and to write up and share the findings. Emphasis needs to be on gathering information within a reasonable length of time and thinking about the implications of the findings for planning interventions.

Although it is difficult to collect information in humanitarian settings, there are some valuable examples that show that it is possible to document sensitive problems such as sexually transmitted infections and sexual violence.[1]

REVIEW OF EXISTING DATA

Before you begin gathering new information it is important to review what already exists. UNAIDS has up-to-date information about prevalence of HIV in different countries (*www.unaids.org*). Bear in mind that the prevalence may vary within a country — and may be different among displaced people. Useful national health, social, and economic data is also available in WHO, UNICEF, and World Bank publications and the UNDP Human Development Report.

Search for other sources of information. Relevant studies may have been published from the same country or region. IRC has published a series of "Lessons learned" reports and "How-to guides" on reproductive health in refugee/IDP situations (see "Additional Resources" below, page 63). Studies of STI prevalence, reproductive health, and surveys of knowledge, attitudes, and practice may all be useful. You can search the Medline and AIDSline databases if you have access to the Internet (available at *www.ncbi.nlm.nih.gov* or *www.medscape.com/*). AIDSline has the abstracts from the international AIDS conferences, which can be useful sources of local information. Ask the UN agencies, other NGOs, and local government about relevant studies or surveys. Sometimes students or others have carried out surveys that are gathering dust on a shelf but may provide relevant and useful data. Other sectoral programs such as health, education, or social welfare may have carried out needs assessments that should be reviewed.

National or provincial health departments may have relevant data, for example, on STI surveillance, tuberculosis rates or prenatal care attendance rates. Community health workers, nurses and doctors, pharmacists, family planning workers, and traditional birth attendants

---

1. S. Swiss et al., "Violence against Women during the Liberian Civil Conflict," *Journal of the American Medical Association* 279 (1998): 625–29. See also P. Salignon et al., "Health and War in Congo-Brazzaville," *Lancet* 356 (2000): 1762.

SEXUAL AND GENDER VIOLENCE
AMONG BURUNDIAN REFUGEES IN TANZANIA

IRC has been assisting the Burundi refugees in Tanzania since 1993 and is responsible for primary health care services for the refugees in the Kibondo district. In 1996 IRC began to address the difficult issue of sexual and gender violence, in addition to the existing range of reproductive health services. In the assessment phase of the project IRC staff used group discussions, in-depth interviews, and a community survey of women aged twelve to forty-nine years.

For the in-depth interviews women were invited to come forward at a later time if they were willing to be interviewed. Sixty-eight women were interviewed. The staff found that it was essential that referral services were in place before the assessment so that the immediate needs of the women being interviewed could be met. They found that the group discussions allowed women to describe their experiences, ask questions in the third person, and discuss solutions. They found that using dance and games at the beginning and the end of group discussions helped people to relax and created a friendly, trusting environment.

For the survey they used the camp registry to select every tenth woman to obtain a simple random sample of four hundred women. Eighty-five percent of the women agreed to participate. Women's Representatives, refugees that have been elected by community women to provide leadership, were involved in every step of survey planning and implementation. The questionnaire was translated, back-translated, pre-tested, and modified before use.

The staff believed that the survey was successful because trust had already been built up with the refugees through extensive consultation, and the Women's Representatives conducted the survey. The survey found that about 26 percent of women had experienced sexual violence since becoming a refugee. The qualitative methods gave information about who, where, how, and by whom sexual violence occurred. The staff found that the process of conducting the assessment was very important and led to a determination by the women to see change in the security situation of the camp. The results of the assessment have been used to raise the awareness of camp management, police, UNHCR, and NGO staff, to inform sensitization training and counseling training, and to better manage women who have suffered sexual or gender-based violence.

—Sydia Nduna and Lorelei Goodyear, *Pain Too Deep for Tears: Assessing the Prevalence of Sexual and Gender Violence among Burundian Refugees in Tanzania* (International Rescue Committee, September 1997).

---

may have clinic records or anecdotal information about the pattern and frequency of STIs.

Demographic data describe the composition of a population in terms of age, sex, and socioeconomic and ethnic characteristics. In humanitarian settings this information may be available from registers and assessments conducted during the emergency. But mobility is often a feature of these populations, making it difficult to collect reliable quantitative demographic data. Participatory exercises can be helpful to identify changes in the composition of the population as a result of displacement, current trends, mixing of previously separate populations, and the impact of these changes.

RAPID APPRAISAL OF REPRODUCTIVE HEALTH NEEDS
IN SOUTHERN SUDAN

A study was commissioned by Oxfam to identify reproductive health care needs among a community affected by conflict in southern Sudan. Rapid appraisal methods were used to provide good quality and timely information from local people that would lead directly to interventions. The methods were selected to deliver results in a short time frame, to address sensitive topics, and to be flexible enough to be used in a conflict zone. They used interviews with key informants, in-depth interviews with women, focus group discussions (FGDs), and the collation of secondary data from health facilities, non-governmental sources, and local administrators. The questionnaires and topic guide, based on previous qualitative work on reproductive health, were piloted and revised in the field. The key informants included administrators, leaders, and other authorities; community-based outreach workers; and women from the community. PLA techniques were used to help stimulate discussion during the FGDs. The women were asked to develop lists of illnesses, health care resources, and community priorities, which gave an idea of general awareness of the problems. The women used matrix ranking to rank common diseases and reproductive health problems according to prevalence, impact on the duration of sickness, impact on mortality, and the availability of treatment. The third technique was the use of scenarios in which imaginary stories of an event were presented to the group, who were then asked to describe what the outcome would be if that problem occurred in their own community. One sample scenario concerned pregnancy outside marriage:

"A young girl finds that she is pregnant. She is not married. What is she most likely to do? What else could she do? What will happen to her? What else could happen? What would be a good outcome for the girl? What would be a bad outcome for the girl?" Another concerned domestic violence: "A married woman is being beaten by her husband more and more often. What is the most likely reason that he is beating her? Who will she talk to about her husband? What will she do to try to stop the situation from continuing? What would be a good outcome? What would be a bad outcome for the woman?" In this way sensitive data could be obtained without women having to talk about their own experiences. The group discussions were taped in the field and transcribed later, while interviews were written down in full at the time.

The team was able to carry out twenty interviews with key informants, fourteen in-depth interviews, and twenty-three group discussions within six weeks. Three months after the work was started they were able to prepare a report of the findings. Four main themes were identified:

a. there were clear needs in reproductive health;

b. there was a mismatch between the views of service providers and the community;

c. there was variation in the perception of need according to age, sex, and whether the community was settled or displaced; and

d. there were a lack of supplies and numerous barriers to accessing services.

The study provided useful results and insights that could be used to plan effective reproductive health services.

—Celia A. Palmer, "Rapid Appraisal of Needs in Reproductive Health Care in Southern Sudan: Qualitative Study," *British Medical Journal* 319 (September 18, 1999): 743–48; also available at *http://bmj.com/cgi/content/full/319/7212/743.*

QUANTITATIVE METHODS

Studies of HIV prevalence

The pattern of HIV transmission in populations that have been forced to migrate is likely to differ from that in stable settings. Even in countries that have a generalized epidemic there may be subpopulations with higher rates of HIV. Where resources are very scarce and lives depend on how they are allocated there is an obligation on humanitarian agencies to make rational and well-informed decisions, so it is important to determine the extent and patterns of spread of HIV.

Sentinel surveillance

It is not necessary to test everyone in a country or area to get a good picture of the extent of spread of HIV infection. It is more cost-effective to choose specific groups from which samples are tested intermittently to build up a picture. This is called sentinel surveillance — but is often impossible in humanitarian settings. Sentinel surveillance testing is anonymous and unlinked, and is performed on blood tests taken for other purposes. This means that blood specimens, after other tests have been performed, have all identifying information removed from them and are then tested for HIV antibodies. No one is able to tell who the HIV-positive specimens have come from and people are not informed of the result. This minimizes participation bias. It is also the only ethical way to undertake surveillance testing.

Sentinel groups for surveillance may be representative of the general population, such as pregnant women or blood donors, or representative of vulnerable groups, such as injecting drug users, clients of sex workers, or patients attending STI clinics. The value of prenatal clinic data for HIV surveillance depends on how well pregnant women who attend ANC represent the general population. Selection biases may change over time, making it difficult to interpret trends.

Cross-sectional surveys

Sentinel surveillance is likely to be difficult in most humanitarian settings because it relies on a functioning and accessible health care system. Trends in infection are difficult to measure unless the composition of the groups that are sampled remains stable; obviously this is rare in refugee/IDP settings except in some long-term camps.

In circumstances like these, cross-sectional population-based surveys can give vital information.[2] The same type of cluster sampling methodology that is used to gather other vital quantitative health data rapidly in humanitarian settings can be used. This might be tied in with a survey of STIs. For example, blood may be taken for syphilis serology with the informed consent of the participants in the survey. The blood could then have all identifying information removed before testing for HIV (anonymous unlinked testing). Alternatively the people in the randomly selected sample could be asked if they would be willing to give an anonymous blood or saliva specimen for the purposes of gathering information about the prevalence of HIV. This is called voluntary anonymous testing. The drawback with this approach is that some of the sample may not wish to take part, either because they want to know their HIV test result, or because they do not trust that their name and result will not somehow be linked and confidentiality breached. Regardless of the method used, the study population should be offered voluntary counseling and testing (see chapter 8).

A rapid cross-sectional survey can be carried out among a sample of pregnant women to determine the prevalence of HIV in a population. With rapid test kits such a survey requires little manpower and can be carried out reasonably quickly and cheaply. Do not undertake this without seeking the advice of an epidemiologist, through WHO, CDC, UNAIDS, or another appropriate agency. It is important to be aware of the political dangers there may be in such an exercise, and of the need for attention to confidentiality in unstable settings.

Notification of AIDS cases

Information on the number of AIDS cases in a population is not useful for assessing the size

2. P. Salama, T. Dondero, "HIV Surveillance in Complex Emergencies," *AIDS* 15, suppl. 3 (2001): S4–S12.

of the problem or trends in the spread of the epidemic, because the cases reported represent HIV infection acquired years earlier.

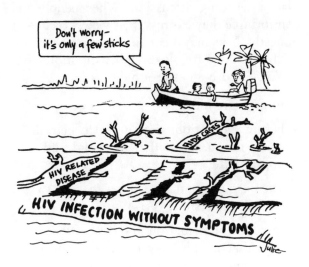

Also, AIDS may remain undiagnosed or unreported. Clinic or admission data on numbers of patients with AIDS may be useful for planning and developing services for the treatment and care of people with the disease.

Data from voluntary counseling and testing services

Unlinked testing is different from voluntary named testing, when people do receive their results, which should always be accompanied by counseling. When voluntary named testing is offered there will always be some people who do not want to be tested. Voluntary testing services are important for HIV prevention and care (see page 87) but are not useful for the purpose of surveillance. It is important to understand that the results from voluntary testing services and from cases reported by doctors cannot give information about rates of HIV in the population. This is because those tested are not representative of the population, or of groups within the population.

Mandatory testing

In refugee/IDP settings there are sometimes calls for mandatory or compulsory testing for HIV. It is important to understand the difference between anonymous unlinked testing for surveillance purposes and mandatory testing. In mandatory testing persons are tested for HIV

without their informed consent, and the result is linked to their name. The result may be used to discriminate against them in some way; for example, they may be isolated, denied consideration for resettlement, or refused surgery or other medical attention. Compulsory testing breaches human rights and does not help to prevent the spread of HIV.

Questionnaire surveys

Questionnaire surveys can provide reliable information about the magnitude of a problem or the level of knowledge, attitudes, and behaviors in a population. However, they take time and require expertise to carry out properly. It is unwise to plan a community questionnaire survey unless you have someone on the team who is familiar with sampling methods and questionnaire design and analysis.

Planning

Survey planning includes the following steps:

- consult and gather background information,
- define the study population,
- obtain permission from appropriate institutions (e.g., government, UNHCR),
- select appropriate sample size and sampling method,
- design and pre-test questionnaire,
- estimate time needed and costs,
- consider ethical issues, including informed consent and confidentiality,
- select and train interviewers.

Sampling

A suitable sampling method for rapid community surveys involves two hundred to three hundred household interviews, drawn from thirty clusters of seven to ten respondents each. The method is described in detail in "Module 2 — Assessing Community Health Needs and Coverage" of the Primary Health Care Management Advancement Programme (PHCMAP) of the Aga Khan Health Network. This is a particularly useful guide to rapid community surveys. It is available in PDF format at *http://erc.msh.org/toolkit/map.htm* or in text and WordPerfect formats at *www.jhsph.edu.*

Epi-info is a statistical software program designed to help to analyze questionnaire surveys. It is available free at *www.cdc.gov* along with a training guide.

Bias

The goal of a quantitative survey is to produce accurate statistics, but several sources of bias, or error, may affect the results. The sample may not be representative of the whole population. The way the sample is chosen, and the size of the sample, affect how well it represents a population. Some in the sample may decline to take part, or cannot be contacted. The questionnaire may include questions that are not clear or mean different things to different people. Different interviewers may ask the questions in different ways or in a different order so that they get different answers. People interviewed may be embarrassed or fearful to answer sensitive questions honestly, or they may not remember events accurately if asked to recall over a long period. Errors may also occur when the results are tallied or entered into a computer.

Guides for questionnaire surveys

- *Health Research Methodology: A Guide for Training in Research Methods.* WHO, 1992.
- Nichols, Paul. *Social Survey Methods.* Oxfam Development Guidelines 6. Oxfam Publishing.
- "Refugee Reproductive Health Needs Assessment Field Tools 1997." Refugee Reproductive Health Consortium. *www.rhrc.org.*
- Vaughan, J. P., and R. H. Morrow. *Manual of Epidemiology for District Health Management.* Geneva: WHO, 1989.

QUALITATIVE METHODS

Data Collection Tools

Focus group discussions

A focus group discussion (FGD) is an in-depth discussion in which a small number of people (usually six to ten) from the study population, guided by a trained facilitator, discuss relevant topics. The group dynamics may stimulate interesting discussion. When people feel comfortable they express their views freely and honestly. You may hear information that you might not think to ask about in a questionnaire.

You can use focus group discussions:

- to generate ideas;
- before a questionnaire survey to help in choosing questions that are valid and appropriate;
- after a questionnaire survey to help to explain the results;
- to collect information about sensitive subjects that people may not answer in a questionnaire or interview;
- to pre-test messages and IEC materials;
- to assist in the design of interventions and program planning;
- in evaluation, to describe changes in knowledge, attitudes, and behaviors.

The discussion should take place in a setting that is comfortable, private, and familiar to the participants, and where there will be few interruptions.

The participants are chosen to be representative rather than picked randomly. It is important to consider whether all the different groups of interest are represented — for example, young and old, women and men, rural and urban people — and to think about possible problems. Then consider how to best combine groups so that everyone will be able to discuss openly. For example, young people may be unwilling to give their views in front of elders; young men and young women may not speak freely together.

If possible it is best to tape the discussion. Obtain permission from the participants first. Ensure secure storage of the tapes afterward so that they cannot be misused. People may be identified by their voices or the things that they say. If a tape recorder is not available, try to have two people who are able to write quickly and accurately to take notes. It is also helpful to take notes about the atmosphere of the group discussion and record when people were joking or solemn.

The facilitator should talk to participants before the discussion to assure that they understand the purpose of the discussion, to ask them to sign a consent form (if appropriate), and to explain that they are free to leave at any time if they wish to.

When people are sitting comfortably the facilitator introduces the discussion by explaining the reason for gathering the information and asking that everyone keep what is said in the discussion confidential.

Facilitators usually begin the discussion with general issues and then move on to more specific issues. The facilitators try to draw out the quieter participants and to prevent any one from dominating the discussion. They need to provide a supportive atmosphere and listen well. With sensitive issues they need to watch for signs that someone is upset. The facilitators need to be trained and to have a chance to practice facilitating discussions.

The discussion continues until everyone has said all that they want to say about the topics. This will usually be about one hour.

There is no rule about how many FGDs to have. Usually after two or three discussions you find that you are hearing the same points and that more FGDs do not produce any additional information. FGDs should be held with each subgroup of the study population, for example, with both sexes, or young and old.

FGDs may be a culturally appropriate means to gather information. In many societies it is traditional to discuss problems in a group to reach solutions.

People do not always talk freely in a focus group discussion, especially when the topic is sensitive or personal (see page 50). When participatory learning and action (PLA) exercises are used in a focus group discussion people often find it easier to talk because they do not have to look at each other. They can also talk about the experiences of their peers rather than their own. But for very sensitive topics such as sexual abuse a confidential one-to-one interview may be more appropriate.

In-depth interviews

General information on community knowledge, attitudes, beliefs, and practices related to HIV/AIDS can be gathered from in-depth interviews with a range of community members (key informant interviews). These are confidential one-to-one interviews using a question guide rather than a questionnaire. They generally last for half an hour to one hour. Key informants might include community leaders, teachers, religious leaders, local government leaders, police or military, brothel managers, and the heads of women's groups. People whose occupation enables them to talk with a wide variety of people are also useful informants about behavior and attitudes. These might include bus or auto-rickshaw drivers, hairdressers, market stallholders, those who sell medicines, and café owners. In addition, members of groups perceived to be at high risk (e.g., sex workers, single young men) should be interviewed.

In-depth interviews can be useful for finding out about sensitive subjects, but this is only likely to occur if the person trusts the interviewer. You can obtain more in-depth information from an interview than an FGD or a survey because one person is able to talk for a long time about a particular issue. However, you can obtain the views of more people, more quickly, using FGDs. To obtain the views of the same number of people will take longer with interviews than FGDs. There may be insufficient interviewers, or interviewers may become tired.

Some tips for interviewing:

- Be polite, respectful, and friendly.

- Explain the purpose of the interview in a way that the person you want to interview is able to understand. Ensure that the person has given consent to be interviewed and understands that they can say that they prefer not to answer any question, or can stop the interview at any time.

- Reassure the person that everything said in the interview will be treated confidentially and that their name will not be on the notes.

- Be patient; don't be in a hurry.

- If possible use the same language, and in the same way, as the persons being interviewed. This is important so that they feel comfortable and are able to understand the questions.

- Don't take too much of their time. Try to minimize inconvenience by choosing the time and setting of the interview carefully.

- Respect the privacy of the person being interviewed. Try to prevent interruptions during the interview.

- Be familiar with the question guide. This means that you can be flexible during the interview, without missing important questions.

- Listen carefully; show interest in the person's answers. Be careful not to show disapproval, surprise, or embarrassment at the answers.

- Be confident. If you are nervous the person you are interviewing will feel nervous.

- Ask easy and nonthreatening questions first. Ask the person to introduce himself or herself to you by asking questions such as: "What kind of work do you do?" "Do you have children?" "What is your situation like at home?" Ask questions about attitudes or about sensitive topics later in the interview.

- It can be helpful to ask the person you are interviewing to tell you a story related to the topic, for example, the story of their last pregnancy, or the first time they bought a condom. What were the circumstances? How did they feel?

- Check that the person you are interviewing understands your questions; repeat a question in a different way if they do not understand.

- Use open questions rather than closed questions. A closed question is one that can be answered with a single word — often "yes" or "no." Closed questions tend to stop the conversation.

- Avoid asking leading questions. A leading question is a question that suggests the answer. For example: "Would you go to the clinic or the pharmacy if you had an STI?" Instead use, "If you thought that you had an STI, what would you do and who would you talk to?"

- Ask one question at a time.

- Don't give your own opinion.

- If you do not understand what the person is trying to tell you ask them to try to explain in a different way.

- If the subject is a sensitive one take care to notice if the person you are interviewing becomes upset, embarrassed, or offended.

- If the person you are interviewing shows by their answers that they have important gaps in their knowledge or misconceptions do not correct them during the interview. But at the end of the interview, once you have thanked them, it is appropriate to provide them with the correct facts.

Participatory appraisal exercises

A number of ideas have been developed to enable people to express and share information, to stimulate discussion. They do not depend on literacy. These methods aim to lead to community action through raising awareness and stimulating discussion of responses to problems. This approach has been given several names including "Participatory Learning and Action" (PLA), "Participatory Rural Appraisal" (PRA), and "Participatory Action Research" (PAR). These terms are used in different ways by different people. Some distinguish them depending on the techniques used, others by the setting, or by the aim of the process.

The PLA approach was developed to be an ongoing community development process of sharing information, planning and implementing actions, and evaluation. However, the techniques can also be used simply to facilitate the collection of information in a participatory way. The uncertain and temporary nature of many humanitarian situations may not be conducive to a long-term community development process, but this does not mean that PLA exercises will not be valuable tools in gathering information relevant to sexual health and to HIV prevention and care.

Examples of participatory exercises include:

- **Ranking:** using matrices or grids for comparisons or prioritizing, for example, using the "ten seed technique" (see page 204) showing what proportion of local people or peers have a particular practice, belief, or behavior.

- **Flow diagrams:** showing linkages, causes, effects, problems, and solutions, including "causal diagrams" and "problem trees."

- **Mapping:** showing the location of important local features such as health facilities, markets, schools, clusters of bars or brothels, roads and bridges, and social structures.

- **Seasonal calendar:** showing how food availability, movements, workloads, family health, prices, wages, and other factors vary during the year.

- **Body mapping:** showing through drawings how people understand the structure and function of their body; participants may draw around a member of the group to produce an outline.

- **Time-lines:** showing trends and change over time.

- **Role-plays:** making up scripts and acting out scenarios.

PLA methods are often conducted in an informal way. If carried out in a public space community members are often attracted to join in the discussion so that a wide range of views can be obtained. Of course it is important to consider whether participants are representative of the general community. It is also important to consider how the time of day, the season, and the setting may influence the type of people who are able to participate in the exercise. Check that you have been able to hear the views of different groups of people, for example, women, older people, younger people, and minority groups.

Sometimes a group of people, such as women, or young men, or sex workers, is deliberately invited to take part in PLA exercises. These methods can be very useful within focus group discussions on sensitive subjects. One of the advantages is that eye contact can be avoided because the activity becomes the focus, and people tend to look down at the matrix, map, or diagram on the floor rather than at each other. Participants can talk about what happens in their community or with their peers rather than about their own individual experiences or behaviors.

Appendix C (page 201) has some examples of participatory exercises for gathering information about sensitive issues such as gender and reproductive and sexual health. These are best thought of as a set of tools or ideas. Once you become familiar with them you can move from one to another in the course of a discussion on a topic and make up your own variations.

These techniques depend on good facilitation. It can be difficult to identify people who will be good facilitators. They do not need to be highly educated, but they do need to be confident, yet willing not to dominate a discussion. They have to be able to draw people out and to notice when something interesting is said and be able to follow it up with further relevant questions.

Probing for further information and encouraging discussion rather than simple question-and-answer sessions are important facilitation skills that improve with practice. Facilitators need to be well informed about HIV infection and comfortable when talking about sexual issues.

Observation

Looking and listening can reveal a great deal about the structure and way of life in a refugee/IDP camp or refugee-affected area. It is important for the team to discuss a checklist for observations and to discuss the findings afterward in order to understand their meanings. Through observation you can document information about, for example, how young people prefer to spend their time, how the roles of the sexes differ, and where people gather, that will be relevant to developing interventions.

Planning for qualitative methods

The following steps are helpful in planning:

- decide who will be appropriate participants;

- decide an appropriate venue or setting;

- consider ethical issues;
- prepare a question guide;
- prepare consent forms;
- train facilitators/interviewers and note-takers;
- consider practical details: transport, refreshments, child-care;
- make a checklist of things to take;
- have a pilot or "test" discussion to identify any practical problems or problems with the question guide.

Preparing question guides

It is best to prepare the question guide with the team. Brainstorm a list of questions and then sort the questions into categories or themes. The first question on a topic should be broad so that you find out what the person thinks without suggesting possible answers. After several responses have been given the interviewers or facilitators might prompt "Any other reasons or suggestions?" Then if a particular point of interest has not been mentioned, they might probe further with a leading question. Probes can be written in italics to remind the interviewers or facilitators that they should not be included in the first question — they should only be asked if there is no answer to the broad question or no mention of the particular point of interest. The box on page 49 contains some examples.

The facilitator and interviewer need to be aware there is no strict order for these questions. If something has already been discussed in answer to an earlier question the facilitator should not ask the question — it tends to stop the discussion. This means that the facilitator has to listen well.

Analysis of qualitative data

It is best to analyze the results in a small team. After the discussions and interviews the tapes are transcribed or the notes checked for gaps and consistency. Make two or three photocopies of the text ready for the analysis. Become familiar with the data. Read the notes carefully — then read them again. Discuss interpretation of the data with others. Look for the deeper meanings in what people say. Look for patterns and similarities in people's views. Look for clues about why they have the beliefs, attitudes, or practices that they have. Also look for statements or beliefs that are different from the majority. Discuss with others why they might be different. Take the context of the discussion or interview into account when you analyze the data. This means you should think about the atmosphere of the discussion or interview. Were people serious or laughing? Were people shy or relaxed?

One way to group the statements in the data is to write the topic headings or main question themes as headings on large sheets of paper. Read through the transcripts or notes together, cut out what people say and decide where the comment or story belongs. It might belong in more than one category. Stick the quotes to the large sheets of paper. If a new idea or point is made, write a new heading. In this way new themes come from what people have said. When all the transcripts have been cut up, read through the ideas and points under each heading. Discuss the main points and findings and write a summary. It is useful to write down direct quotes that illustrate the points well.

Capturing and analyzing the findings from participatory exercises can present problems. Some of the techniques, such as creating problem trees or causal diagrams, assist in a participatory process of analysis because they investigate underlying causes of problems rather than simply describing how things are. The technique of writing up points made under theme headings on large sheets of paper described above is also helpful. It is difficult for people who are not literate to participate fully in the analysis.

Capturing the findings of PLA exercises requires thought. A beautiful map may be drawn in the sand, illustrated with twigs, seeds, and pebbles, but it will be more useful for planning if it can be captured by being copied onto paper. With other visual techniques such as matrix ranking (see page 47) and the ten seed technique (see page 204), someone, preferably with a talent for drawing, needs to be nominated to make sketches of the outcomes of the participatory work and to make notes of what

EXAMPLE OF PART OF A QUESTION GUIDE (THEME LIST) ABOUT CONDOM USE

The probes are in italics. These should be asked only if they are not covered in the respondent's answer to the question. For an FGD the questions would be better in the third person, e.g., "What are the reasons that people use condoms? What difficulties do people have in obtaining condoms?"

Knowledge about condoms	Can you tell the story of the first time that you heard about condoms? Have you ever been taught how to use a condom? *If so, who taught you?* How do you dispose of condoms? Where can you obtain condoms? How much do condoms cost?
Patterns of condom use	How often do you use a condom? *Is it every time that you have sex?* *Do you use condoms when you have sex with your wife?* Do you use condoms when you have sex outside marriage?
Reasons for using condoms	What are the reasons that you use a condom? *To protect yourself and your partner from sexually transmitted infections/from HIV?* *To protect against pregnancy?* *To reassure your partner?*
Attitudes about condom use	Can you tell me about the things that you like about condoms and the things that you don't like? What does your partner think about using condoms? What are the reasons why you don't use a condom? *Religious beliefs? Can't get them? Uncomfortable?* *Embarrassed? Partner doesn't like them? Want to have a child?* *Forget to have them with you?*
Obstacles to condom use	What difficulties do you find in obtaining condoms? *Too expensive? not available at the shop? too shy to ask?*

people say. The drawings and quotes can be used to illustrate a report of the findings. In some situations capturing participatory exercises and discussions on camera or video might be a possibility, but this may inhibit people who are reluctant to be identified. Making a video requires relatively expensive equipment, electricity, and someone skilled in filming and editing.

Share your findings with members of the refugee, IDP, and local communities to check the meaning and interpretation of results.

Discuss conclusions from the findings. What do the findings mean for your activities? The findings should help you to understand people's attitudes, beliefs, and practices. They should help you to understand the barriers to behavior change and suggest ideas to help people to change risky behaviors. They should help you to decide how to develop effective messages.

ETHICAL CONSIDERATIONS

The aim of collecting information is to be able to plan and carry out better activities to solve problems. But when we collect information we may do harm without meaning to. There is a need to think about the potential for harm at the level of the individual and of the community, so that we can try to avoid it.

Potential harm to individual participants

- *exposure to discrimination (including physical harm) or loss of reputation if confidentiality is breached*

  This can be especially serious in humanitarian settings if people learn, for example, that someone has HIV or an STI, has been raped, or has had a pregnancy terminated.

- *discomfort, embarrassment, or shame*

  We should be aware that during PLA exercises and FGDs an open and trusting environment might be built in which people might say more than they intended. If this information is then shared in a larger group, the person may feel ashamed or embarrassed. When visited to seek their opinions or ask questions, refugees and IDPs may feel self-conscious about their poor surroundings and inability to offer hospitality. It is important to show respect.

- *emotional distress*

  A woman who has been beaten by her husband may become distressed in a focus group discussion if the subject of family violence comes up, or a girl who has been raped or sexually abused may feel bad if she is asked about sexual abuse in an interview. Opinions expressed in a group environment may get people into trouble when they return to the private space of home.

- *fear*

  A boy who admits an illegal activity in an interview, such as injecting drugs, may worry that the police will find out and arrest him or keep a watch on him.

- *offense*

  Lack of knowledge of the local culture may result in offending someone by asking an inappropriate question. During FGDs and interviews it is important not to make assumptions about people's sexual practices and to remember that any member of the group may be infected with HIV.

Potential harm to the community

- *disempowerment, feeling inferior*

  If a study is carried out with the participation of the community at all stages, then it is an empowering process. On the other hand, if the researchers do not consult and do not include the community, then the result can be that the community feels they have been viewed as passive objects. Displaced and conflict-affected communities are already likely to feel powerless, and these feelings can be reinforced.

- *harmful stereotyping*

  This may be especially significant in refugee and IDP communities. "Bad publicity" about levels of HIV, injecting drug use, sexual violence, or sex work may all add to discrimination experienced by refugees, decreasing the willingness of the host government to provide shelter, and of third countries to resettle refugees.

- *disappointment or feeling misled*

  A situation analysis may raise expectations that something will be done about the problems and needs that are identified.

- *feeling drained, overburdened by questions*

  Sometimes communities, or groups within a community, become over-researched. For example, a researcher from the university may carry out a survey among young refugees/IDPs using questionnaires. Next a team from an international aid agency carries out a study using focus group discussions, and then a theater group that is researching a new script for a health promotion play comes to do some in-depth interviews. When the local youth worker starts to do a needs assessment among the young people, they are likely to refuse to take part! In this situation, when people are asked to be in many studies they can feel drained of information and burdened by all the questions.

- *loss of resources, e.g., time, energy, food*

  Communities often have a custom of hospitality and offer food, time, and energy to people who visit to carry out a survey or study. It is important to think of this in the budget. If people are likely to provide hospitality, then it is important to take a suitable gift that will recompense the community.

How to avoid causing harm

Consultation can reduce the chance of harm occurring. There is a need to think about the different groupings in a community and consult widely — not just with one person or group. Consultation should begin as early as possible in the planning process and takes time. The study team and community leaders may prepare a *written agreement* which explains the responsibilities of each and states that they will *share ownership of the data*. Never publish results before discussion with the community.

A small group of people from the community may form an *advisory committee* to advise about the ethical issues in the situation analysis plan.

Community leaders, as well as individual participants and individuals, may need to give *informed consent*. It is important to explain the situation analysis in a way that people can understand. Decide whether oral or written consent will be appropriate. Parents as well as children should give their consent when children are studied. You will need to discuss with the community when young people are old enough not to need parental consent. Take care that each person is able to give free consent and is not feeling coerced into giving consent. In a humanitarian setting individuals should feel reassured that they will not miss out on any services or supplies if they decline to take part.

It is important not only to plan for *confidentiality*, but also to tell participants that all information will be kept confidential. The whole team needs training in the importance of confidentiality. Make sure that others cannot overhear when interviewing, and *store data in a careful, secure, and confidential way*. Questionnaire surveys and qualitative studies should be anonymous. There is no need to take names. If you are undertaking a study that will involve following up with the same people and you need to be able to link the data, then use an identity code rather than the name. Think about *privacy issues* when you plan to use lists of names and addresses. With sensitive topics there is a need for debriefing. An interviewer who hears distressing information needs to be able to talk about it to someone else. An outsider on the team can be useful in this role.

When there is a chance that participants might become upset or humiliated as a result of taking part in an interview or discussion, it is important to be able to *offer supportive counseling*, or just the chance to talk, afterward. Some people may express their distress; others might say nothing. So it is important that the potential for distress is acknowledged at the beginning of the discussion and the offer of counseling support made to all. Other strategies to avoid this harm might be to ensure that there is an opportunity after a focus group discussion for people to undertake some other social activity so that facilitators can notice if someone seems to be upset.

Care should be taken to distinguish between a therapeutic interview or counseling session and a research interview. For example, when information is gathered about depression or sexual violence from women who have experienced these, it should be absolutely clear to both the researcher and the woman whether the aim of the interview is to assist the woman or to gather information. If the aim is to gather information, for example, to develop interventions that will benefit other women, the woman should be aware of this and informed consent should be obtained. If a woman has had no opportunity to talk about her problems before, she may say more than she intends and regret being so open when she realizes that her story is being documented for a report, even if this is done anonymously.

It may be appropriate to make a small payment of money or food to participants, especially if they are losing income by spending time participating. The amount should not be an inducement to take part. It should not be so large that the person takes part only because of the payment.

RESPONSE REVIEW

In addition to understanding the ways that HIV spreads within the community, there is also a need to understand and analyze what has and is being done to reduce risk and support those infected and affected by the virus. This should include an assessment of what programs and services are being implemented, who is doing this, whether the programs and services are working well, and where there are gaps. Asking about relevant existing programs provides an opportunity to raise the morale of those involved but has the potential to undermine the workers' confidence if done insensitively. It is helpful to assess the services and program activities from the perspective of groups within the community (mothers, sex workers, young people, men) and of the providers. Putting these perspectives together may reveal important gaps and opportunities to improve services.

PRESENTING THE FINDINGS

The findings will need to be presented in a way that different audiences will be able to understand. The community should receive feedback about the results of the situation analysis. The findings also need to be shared with other stakeholders such as the local government departments, the UN agencies, and other international and national NGOs.

Prepare a written report with a summary of the key findings, as well as the detailed findings from the analysis. The quantitative data will be illustrated with tables and graphs. Keep these simple. Avoid three-dimensional shaded representations of data just because this feature is available on the computer. Simple outline pie charts and histograms are clear and easiest to understand. The key points from the qualitative data should be illustrated with verbatim quotes. Consider preparing a shorter community report in simple language that can be easily translated, with drawings and photographs taken during the situation analysis. Remember to check for permission from the people pictured before you make copies. The community report can be a useful information and communication tool.

These reports might be distributed through community groups and buildings and at the strategic planning meeting. Remember that your findings may well be relevant to workers in other parts of the country or region. After seeking necessary approval you might consider putting the information on the Internet or sending an article to a relevant journal or newsletter.

GUIDE FOR PLANNING THE SITUATION ANALYSIS AND RESPONSE REVIEW

At a workshop to plan the situation analysis work through the following questions:

- Who will participate in the situation analysis team?

- Within the team who will perform what roles?

- How long will you allow for the situation analysis? (This will depend on the scope of the exercise. It may take from a few weeks to several months.)

- In which sites will you select samples?

- Who will you consult with?

- Who will be responsible for reviewing the existing data?

- Who could be useful key informants for in-depth interviews?

- What topics would you ask about with the different key informants?

- Who will interview the key informants?

- Will additional technical help be needed?

- What focus group discussions will you carry out?

- Who will be the participants (type, age, gender)?

- How many focus group discussions do you think you will carry out on the different topics? How will you group the topics?
- Where will you hold the FGDs (in a home, a school or clinic, etc.)?
- When will you hold the FGDs? What time of day?
- What costs will be involved? Prepare a budget under the following headings:
  - Preparation costs (further planning and practice)
  - Transport
  - Stationery
  - Equipment, e.g., hire of tape recorder, tapes
  - Refreshments and/or payments for FGD participants/interviewees
  - Meeting costs to discuss progress and findings (monitor and evaluate)

Draw a timeline showing the weeks of the time period you have agreed to on large sheets of paper and stick them on a wall. Put your plans into the timeline. Remember that it always takes longer than you think to analyze and write up the findings.

- Does it all fit?
- Do you have enough workers?
- Do you have enough time?
- Do you have enough money?

If not, you need to prioritize and/or obtain more resources. Decide what it is most important to do. Cut down on your plans. Don't be too ambitious. Think about how you will use the information. But keep the original plans — perhaps you can come back to them later when you have more resources! Or perhaps you will get on better than you think.

6

The Strategic Planning Process

Ideally the strategic planning process will be multisectoral, including representatives of all the groups who work with and have responsibilities in relation to the beneficiaries, as well as representatives of the beneficiary population themselves. Refugee and IDP settings differ in many ways from permanent communities. In these settings it may be difficult to know what "community participation" means. It is important to understand the structure of the refugee/IDP camp or resettling population. Responsibilities are often divided between different organizations. There may be many groups to include: national and local levels of the host government, local refugee/IDP leaders (including traditional chiefs, religious leaders, and civil or military leaders), local NGOs, international NGOs, church groups, UNHCR and other UN agencies, local military, and UN military. In refugee and IDP-affected areas the host population may resent the displaced. There may be tensions between groups and, despite good intentions, coordination and communication between the different players may be poor.

Some of the stakeholders may not be convinced of the need to address the issue of HIV prevention and care. Inviting them to a strategic planning session may raise their awareness of the vulnerability of the population and the potential severity of the impact of the epidemic. For many displaced and conflict-affected populations HIV will not be a priority, compared to the daily struggle for survival. But other consequences of unsafe sex — unwanted pregnancies, STIs, and infertility — are often issues of great concern. Addressing these issues will also help to prevent the spread of HIV.

Depending on what has already happened it may be appropriate to invite everyone to a preliminary strategic planning meeting. At this meeting the findings of the situation analysis would be considered, priority areas and broad objectives determined. Then smaller working groups could be identified to take responsibility for more detailed planning in specific areas for particular groups.

It is easy for discussions about HIV infection to go off at a tangent. It will be helpful to structure the planning sessions carefully. A useful tip is to have a wide bowl filled with sand and some twigs with paper "flags" stuck on. When someone asks a question or makes an interesting point that is not related to the current discussion it is written on one of the "flags" and stuck in the sand. At the end of the session the flags are read out and any ideas or questions that have not been covered can be dealt with.

GUIDING PRINCIPLES

In the first session of the meeting you might decide to brainstorm a list of principles that will guide your planning. These might include commitment to:

- a human-rights perspective;
- recognition that vulnerability to HIV is determined not only by individual behaviors but also by the societal context and by the coverage and quality of services;
- intersectoral planning and implementation;
- participatory processes (including men, women, youth, and people living with HIV in gathering information, planning, implementation, and evaluation);
- integration with existing activities;
- equality of access to prevention and care services and activities for refugees, IDPs, and host populations;
- consistency with national AIDS control programs, policies, and plans;

- planning based on local situation analysis and published research;

- recognition of the importance of analyzing gender roles of men and women, the relations between them, and the impact of displacement on these — ensuring activities both assist men and women in their gender roles and foster gender equity;

- recognition of the uncertain and often temporary nature of the humanitarian situation and the need to plan flexible activities with short-term outcomes as well as longer-term goals;

- coordination, communication, and collaboration between organizations;

- enabling people with HIV to live productive and positive lives; taking the reduction of stigma and discrimination as a cross-cutting issue;

- recognition of the importance of linking prevention with nondiscriminatory care and support;

- identifying and working with community members previously trained in skills relevant to HIV prevention, e.g., IEC, media, counseling;

- interventions that are feasible;

- ongoing documentation and dissemination of lessons learned.

DEFINING THE PROBLEMS AND GAPS IN THE RESPONSE

It can be helpful to have the main problems that were identified during the situation analysis written on cards. Cut out plenty of long, short, and curved arrows from scrap paper. The strategic planning group can lay out the problems joined by arrows to show how they are related.

They can then identify priority areas to address, such as:

- care for people living with HIV/AIDS;

- mitigating the impact on people infected and affected by HIV/AIDS;

- care and support for orphans and other vulnerable children;

- reducing the vulnerability of young people;

- preventing transmission through sex;

- providing a safe blood supply;

- promoting safer drug-injecting behavior;

- preventing transmission in health care settings;

- preventing transmission from parent to child;

- promoting a supportive ethical, legal, and human rights environment.[1]

Working groups can be nominated to take responsibility for suggesting interventions to address the priority areas.

CHOOSING INTERVENTIONS

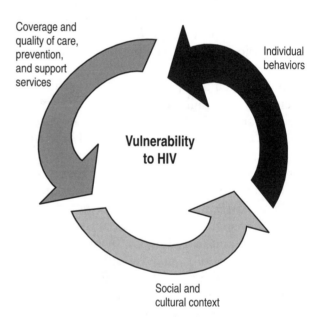

Coverage and quality of care, prevention, and support services

Individual behaviors

Vulnerability to HIV

Social and cultural context

Interventions are needed to address each of these areas of vulnerability.

Vulnerability to HIV

This model of vulnerability presents a useful framework for thinking about interventions. For example, interventions to prevent sexual

---

1. Adapted from *UNAIDS Guide to the Strategic Planning Process for a National Response to HIV/AIDS*, May 1999.

A HUMAN-RIGHTS FRAMEWORK

In recent years much progress has been made in linking the fields of public health and human rights.[2] International documents, such as the Universal Declaration of Human Rights and the Convention Relating to the Status of Refugees define civil, political, economic, social, and cultural rights for all women, men, and children, based on the central importance of human dignity and equality. Increased involvement of civilians in conflicts has reemphasized the need to protect the rights of refugees/IDPs.[3] When human rights are abused HIV has opportunities to spread more easily. Too often strategies to prevent the spread of HIV aim to alter the behavior of individuals and fail to take into account sufficiently the societal factors that determine vulnerability. Jonathan Mann, a leader in the field of health and human rights, compared the disease-inducing effect of violations of dignity with that of bacteria and viruses.

- A human rights framework can help to generate new creative ways to address the spread and impact of HIV.

  For example, efforts to restore displaced persons' rights to dignity will also reduce their vulnerability to spread of HIV and STIs. Social activities can restore dignity, morale, a sense of trust, and hope for the future, can promote equality and respect, and can facilitate companionship, comfort, and consensual sex. They should not be viewed as secondary to the essentials of shelter, water, and food. In camp settings men often lack meaningful activity, which undermines their dignity and is a danger to the physical and mental health of both men and women. Organizing and contributing to social activities and events can provide work as well as entertainment.

- A human rights framework can help us consider how HIV prevention and care activities can contribute to the protection and promotion of rights.

  For example, participatory approaches to HIV prevention and care contribute to the promotion and protection of refugees' and IDPs' rights to self-determination, confidentiality, privacy, information and nondiscrimination. Insistence on voluntary rather than mandatory HIV testing is a more effective public health strategy—but also, importantly, protects these rights.

- A human rights framework can help to avoid unintended consequences of HIV prevention activities for the rights of individuals.

  For example, routine testing for HIV in prenatal clinics may have consequences for the human rights of men as well as women. The majority of infected pregnant women have been infected by their husbands, so a positive HIV test result is often a "marker" of HIV infection in the husband. The woman is put in a position where she has a responsibility to inform her husband of her infection, yet he has not had the opportunity to receive pre-test counseling and give informed consent to knowing his HIV status. A possible solution to this conflict of rights is to encourage, as a routine, that the second prenatal visit be a "couple visit."

---

2. J. Mann et al., "Health and Human Rights," *Health and Human Rights* 1 (1994): 6–23.
3. C. Bruderlein and J. Leaning, "New Challenges for Humanitarian Protection," *British Medical Journal* 319 (1999): 430–35.

transmission of HIV might be considered under the following headings:

Interventions that relate to provision of services

- strengthening of STI management and control;

- condom promotion and distribution;

- establishment and promotion of VCT services.

Interventions that relate to changing individual behaviors

- development and dissemination of communication materials for behavior change;

- peer education (for example, among youth; in the workplace; among married women; among sex workers);

- sex education in schools;

- education by HIV-positive people to reduce discriminatory attitudes and behaviors and stimulate individuals to protect themselves;

- prevention counseling for STI patients.

Interventions that relate to the societal context

- protecting against sexual violence;

- providing opportunities for social activities;

- supporting microfinance programs and income-generating activities;

- supporting meaningful activities and support groups;

- changing community attitudes.

DETAILED PLANNING

Next detailed planning needs to occur to:

- identify specific objectives for each intervention;

- identify the groups that will be involved;

- determine the activities and tasks that will be needed to achieve the objectives;

- decide what resources will be needed;

- prepare a feasible timeline or implementation schedule;

- decide the responsibilities of those involved; and

- formulate a plan for monitoring and evaluation.

The IRC has adopted the "causal pathway" for planning, which has five components. The pathway names the logical steps between what a program will provide and do (Inputs and Activities) and what is expected to happen as a result (Outputs, Effects, and Impact). Some funding agencies use a similar logical planning framework but use different terms, which can be confusing.

In addition to thinking about the logical sequence — or causal pathway — to the desired goals or impacts it is important to consider what might help or hinder the planned activities, how the context may change, and what unintended effects, adverse or beneficial, might result from activities.

In humanitarian settings it is obviously important to incorporate flexibility, and to realize that even more urgent priorities may arise. Possible changes in the context need to be considered and plans made to respond to them. These can be described in a "risk matrix" — a grid with columns for "risk," "probability," "likely impact," and "action to minimize or respond to the risk."

PLANNING FOR MONITORING AND EVALUATION

What do we mean by monitoring and evaluation?

Monitoring and evaluation is the process through which we gain information about the activities and achievements of programs in order to make decisions to improve them.[4]

During an evaluation we ask:

- Did we do what we said we were going to do?

- Did we achieve what we said we would achieve?

---

4. *IRC Guide to Program Planning and Proposal Development: Effective Design, Monitoring, and Evaluation of IRC Projects Field Operations Manual* and *The Training Guide to IRC's Program Design, Monitoring, and Evaluation Framework* (New York: IRC and Columbia University, Joseph L. Mailman School of Public Health, 2000).

THE CAUSAL PATHWAY

Component	Description	Alternative names
Inputs	Resources needed to support the activities	Resources Costs
Activities	Technical and support tasks required to produce the output	Tasks Throughputs
Outputs	Products and services that must be in place for the effects and impact on the population of interest to occur	Results
Effects	Change in the knowledge, attitudes, skills, and/or behavior of the population of interest that contribute to the desired impact	Purpose Immediate objectives
Impact	Change in the health, social, economic status of the population of interest	Goal Development objective

---

- Was the planning sound? How can it be improved?

- What was the impact of changes in the context since the plans were first made?

- Did we respond appropriately to these changes?

- Were there unintended consequences — beneficial or adverse?

- Did our activities cause the observed change?

- What other factors contributed to the effects and impacts?

- What now needs to be modified?

There is also a need to evaluate crosscutting issues such as gender, management, ethics, and equity of access. In humanitarian settings where the context may change in unpredictable ways there is an even greater need for ongoing monitoring of plans and regular evaluation.

There are many resources that deal with the important topic of evaluation in more depth than we are able to in this manual. In particular you could review the *IRC Guide to Program Planning and Proposal Development: Effective Design, Monitoring, and Evaluation of IRC Projects in the Field Operations Manual* and *The Training Guide to IRC's Program Design, Monitoring, and Evaluation Framework*. The manual *National AIDS Programmes: A Guide to Monitoring and Evaluation* has a useful discussion of a wide range of indicators for measuring the process and impact of HIV prevention and care interventions.[5]

Timing of evaluation

A plan for monitoring and evaluation should include the timing of evaluation sessions. This will be influenced by the implementation timetable and the players involved. It may be that the different groups responsible for different priority areas will each undertake their own monitoring and evaluation. However, regular meetings for communication, coordination, and monitoring will facilitate the needed integration of activities. Practical factors, such as

---

5. UNAIDS, *National AIDS Programmes: A Guide to Monitoring and Evaluation*, MEASURE Evaluation (June 2000). Available at *www.cpc.unc.edu*.

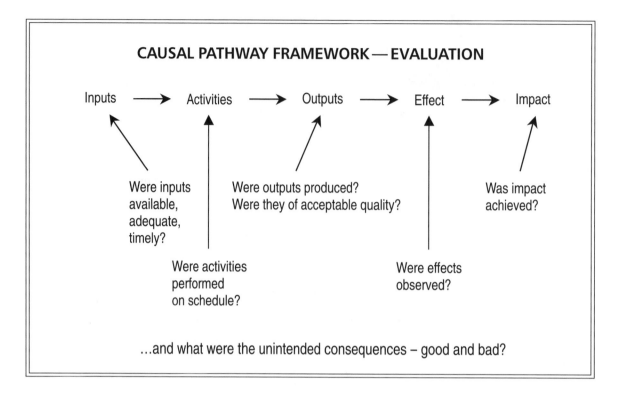

when staff and community can give time to evaluation, also need to be considered. For example, if you plan an evaluation at harvest time it will be difficult for the local community to be involved. Remember to budget for the evaluation.

Indicators

Indicators are signals or measures that indicate progress toward the planned goals or impacts. You can choose indicators to measure progress at different stages along the "causal pathway."

Output indicators

Output indicators measure products and services and their quality. For example:

- number of clinic staff trained in counseling;

- percentage of trained clinic staff who received a rating of "good" or "excellent" on final training exercise.

Output indicators are directly related to activities and can usually be quickly and easily measured. But output indicators do not measure or indicate whether you have achieved your planned goal or impact.

Effect indicators

Indicators of effect measure changes in behavior, knowledge, attitudes, skills, or intentions of the population of interest. For example:

- percentage of sexually active young people who state that they used a condom during their last sexual encounter;

- increase in confidence of young people attending a youth center;

- number of people living with HIV who attend a support group.

Effect indicators show changes in people's behavior, skills, or beliefs, and may be adequate if the link between the effect and the impact is clear and strong. However, they do not measure the impact of interventions and do not indicate what has caused the change. Effect indicators may be qualitative or quantitative. Quantitative measures of effect usually require surveys that can be difficult and expensive to undertake.

Impact indicators

Impact indicators measure the status of the population of interest. For example:

- prevalence of HIV;

- prevalence of STIs;

- infant mortality rate.

Changes in impact rates and ratios usually occur slowly and can be difficult, or impossible, to measure. They are more likely to be measured at a provincial or national level.

Impact indicators will reveal whether you achieved the planned goal. However, there may have been many influences that affected the outcome. Change may have occurred because of the planned activities or may have been influenced by some change in the context. Similarly the status of the population may have been adversely affected by factors unrelated to your activities.

In places with a major HIV epidemic, the impact of the epidemic may make it increasingly difficult to implement effective services — for example, because they become overwhelmed by patients and resources become exhausted, while service providers fall ill and die. In such cases, it may be difficult to show that an intervention is working, as impact indicators may worsen during the project period even though project interventions are having some beneficial effects. The evaluation report may then argue that services might have degenerated even more without the support of the project.

Choosing indicators

How far along the pathway you measure will depend on:

- how strong the links are between the components of the causal pathway;

- what changes are likely to be observable given the time frame, the starting point, and the likely pace of change;

- methodological constraints;

- political/policy/cultural constraints; and

- the resources available.

Do not choose too many indicators. Think about what best represents what you are trying to achieve, and measure or describe that. It is tempting to list every indicator that you can think of to show that you have thought of everything. You do not need to be comprehensive.

You also need to think for each indicator how it will be measured, described, or verified. Indicators are often quantitative, but it is also useful to have some qualitative, or descriptive, indicators.

For some interventions it is best to avoid choosing indicators that rely on reports, such as "decreased clinic reports of STI cases," "decreased reports of needle-stick injuries and blood exposures by health care staff" or "decreased reports of sexual violence." This is because trends in these reports will depend on:

- the quality of the service;

- access to the services;

- awareness of the population;

- willingness to attend with an STI or after being raped;

- the quality of recording of consultations; as well as

- the actual rate of incidents of sexual violence or STI in the community.

Your programs are likely to increase the quality and accessibility of services, raise awareness in the community, and improve reporting, as well as prevent the problems. So rates of reported cases of STIs, needle-stick incidents, and sexual violence would be likely to increase at first. It is important to document reported rates of STIs, needle-stick incidents, and sexual violence, but such statistics need to be interpreted cautiously, and in the light of other information from focus group discussions and community-based surveys.

For each indicator ask:

- Can we measure or describe this indicator before and after the activity or intervention? Will there be sufficient time and resources to do this?

- Does the indicator measure what we are most interested in? Will it contribute information for decision-making?

- Is the indicator valid, that is, does the indicator measure what it is supposed to measure?

- Is the indicator reliable, that is, can it be measured consistently over time by different people? For example, if two outreach workers judge a clinic's adherence to universal precautions guidelines using a checklist, they should both come up with the same rating. To be reliable, an indicator needs to be defined in a specific way.

- Is it possible to measure a change in the indicator within the time period that we can measure it?

If the answer to any of these questions is "no," or "not sure," then cross the indicator off the list.

In this manual we suggest some indicators and a method of measurement or description for each intervention described. These lists of indicators are not intended to be comprehensive and need to be tailored to the circumstances.

If activities and their expected effects and impact are clearly defined, then it is easier to formulate specific indicators that incorporate targets. It is often said that indicators should be SMART—that is:

Specific

Measurable

Appropriate

Reliable, and

Time-bound.

For example: "Percentage of sexually active young people who state that they used a condom during their last sexual encounter increased from 10 percent to 50 percent in two years."

Information gathered in the situation analysis provides a useful baseline against which to measure and describe change. The findings of a baseline survey can also be helpful in deciding the feasibility of indicators. If something was difficult to measure in a baseline survey then it is unlikely to be a useful indicator. If you set targets that are too difficult to achieve, the project team will become discouraged, and

the local community will be disappointed. If baseline measures are available these can help the planning team to set realistic targets. Many variables may be measured during a situation analysis but there may be insufficient time to measure all these variables again. Sometimes it is discovered that the baseline information was unreliable or not precise enough to allow comparisons over time.

Participation

Often staff and community representatives take little part in the monitoring and evaluation process. If the situation analysis has developed participatory processes, there is much more chance that monitoring and evaluation will follow the same processes. Planning and evaluation jargon may make people feel that they cannot understand what it is all about. Evaluation is often perceived as boring, difficult, and complex.

It is possible to make evaluation and monitoring interesting and fun. Staff can keep journals to record thoughts, suggestions, stories, or ideas. Have regular meetings to reflect on progress and difficulties and to talk about the lessons learned. Make these social occasions. You might create a wall newspaper and encourage people to add their own stories. Visual images of progress toward a target can be displayed on walls — for example, a winding road with milestones along it — on which staff and community members can attach stories, photographs, and drawings.

Just as it is essential to take gender into account in planning it is important to evaluate from different perspectives — men and women, old and young. If feasible a video camera can be a useful evaluation tool that can capture the perspectives of men and of women. A group of women can be invited to "direct" a video film — showing the features of their life that are problems or strengths and that have relevance to vulnerability to HIV and their ability to respond. Men could be invited to direct their own film from their perspective. Focus group discussions could also be filmed (with consent of the participants). After an interval the women could be filmed again — watching and discussing their earlier film. It is easy to forget what changes have occurred, but the film can be a reminder of how things were, and what attitudes and knowledge were like before the interventions. Men and women could also watch the films "directed" by the opposite sex.

There is a lot of scope for thinking up new and creative ideas for evaluation. Sensitive subjects are often difficult to document for fear that they will become public knowledge. An example of a creative evaluation idea comes from a project in Nepal in which sex workers were trained as peer educators.[6] Color codes were chosen to represent different outcomes of a sexual encounter — such as "asked to use a condom and agreed," "asked to use a condom and did not agree," "educated client about HIV," and so on. The sex worker peer educators added the appropriately colored bead to their necklace each time that they had an interaction with a client. They ended up with a visual representation of their achievements that no one could understand except the other peer educators. This idea could be adapted for other types of sensitive or confidential activities such as counseling.

ADDITIONAL RESOURCES

Chambers, R. *Rural Appraisal: Rapid, Relaxed, and Participatory.* 1992. FSRC 1988. Outlines the principles, approaches, methods, techniques, and applications of RRA (Rapid Rural Appraisal) and PRA (Participatory Rural Appraisal). Examines the strengths and weaknesses of PRA.

———. *Whose Reality Counts? Putting the First Last.* 1997. Analyzes PRA methodology. Includes theoretical discussion, comparison of PRA and RRA, practical applications, insights from the PRA experience.

Feuerstein, M.-T. *Partners in Evaluation: Evaluating Development and Community Programs with Participants.* London: Macmillan, 1986.

International Institute for Environment and Development. *PLA Notes:* no. 23: "Participatory Approaches to HIV programs"; no. 37: "Sexual and Reproductive Health" (February 2000); e-mail: *iiedagri @gn.apc.org*

Jayakaran, R. *Networking Patterns: Using PLA for Obtaining Sensitive Information.* World Vision of India, undated. Focuses on using PLA techniques for obtaining HIV-related information.

Johnson, D. *Program against Sexual Violence, Congo-Brazzaville.* IRC/UNDP/UNIFEM, January 1999.

Khaw, A. J., et al. "HIV Risk and Prevention in Emergency-Affected Populations: A Review." *Disasters* 24 (September 2000): 181–97.

Manderson, L., and P. Aaby. "An Epidemic in the Field? — Rapid Assessment Procedures and Health Research." *Social Science and Medicine* 35 (1992): 839–50.

Nduna, S., and L. Goodyear. *Pain Too Deep for Tears: Assessing the Prevalence of Sexual and Gender Violence among Burundian Refugees in Tanzania.* New York: International Rescue Committee, September 1997.

Nduna, S., and D. Rude. *A Safe Space Created by and for Women: Sexual and Gender Based Violence Program Phase II Report.* International Rescue Committee, Kibondo, Tanzania. March 1998.

Pratt, B., and P. Loizos. *Choosing Research Methods: Data Collection for Development Workers.* Oxford: Oxfam Publications, 1992.

Pretty, J., et al., *A Trainer's Guide for Participatory Learning and Action.* London: International Institute for Environment and Development, 1995.

Rapid Assessment and Response Guide on Injecting Drug Use (IDU-RAR). Geneva: WHO, 1998. Available from WHO/PSA Geneva.

Scrimshaw, S., et al. *HIV/AIDS Rapid Assessment Procedure Manual.* Geneva: World Health Organization/ Global Programme on AIDS, 1991.

UNAIDS, Inter-Parliamentary Union. *Handbook for Legislators on HIV/AIDS, Law and Human Rights.* 1999.

How-to Guides: Reproductive Health in Refugee Situations

Published by International Rescue Committee, New York

Building a Team Approach to the Prevention and Response to Sexual Violence, Kigoma, Tanzania. UNHCR, 1998.

A Community-Based Response on Sexual Violence against Women. Crisis intervention teams, Ngara, Tanzania. UNHCR, 1997.

Reproductive Health Education for Adolescents, N'zerekore, Guinea. February 1998.

Lessons Learned series

Published by International Rescue Committee, New York

Cote d'Ivoire and Ghana: Family Planning and AIDS Programs. Training Evaluation and Transfer to a Local NGO.

---

6. K. Butcher, S. Baral, K. Bista, and R. Adhikary, "A New Approach to Evaluating Peer Education Programmes for Sex Workers," *PLA Notes* 37 (February 2000).

Goodyear, Lorelei. *Azerbaijan: Introducing Family Planning Education. Two Approaches: Women's Groups and Outreach Workers.* October 1996.

———. *Cambodia: Midwife and Traditional Birth Attendant Training Project.* January 1996.

———. *Pakistan: Providing Family Planning and Emergency Obstetric Care to Afghan Refugees.* July 1997.

Thailand: Fostering Community Ownership. IRC's Reproductive Health Program with Karenni Refugees.

Internet Resources

ELDIS website on participatory monitoring and evaluation. *http://nt1.ids.ac.uk/eldis/hot/pme.htm.*

Institute of Development Studies. "The Power of Participation." IDS Policy Briefing Issue 7. August 1996. *www.ids.ac.uk.*

Reproductive Health for Refugees Consortium. "Refugee Reproductive Health Needs Assessment Field Tools 1997." *www.rhrc.org.*

Part 3

WHAT CAN WE DO
TO CONTRIBUTE TO HIV PREVENTION
AND CARE?

Part 3 presents information about strategies and interventions that contribute to HIV prevention and care. Each chapter in this part has an introduction describing the strategy; a rationale section, which presents the arguments and evidence for adopting the approach; a description of some possible strategies and examples of appropriate evaluation indicators, and it concludes with some suggested additional resources.

Chapter 7 deals with counseling for HIV prevention and care, chapter 8 with prevention of HIV transmission through sex, and chapter 9 with prevention of transmission through injecting drug use. Chapter 10 looks at ways to enable people to live positively with HIV.

7

Counseling for HIV Prevention and Care

Counseling is a process that helps people to cope with problems and to make their own decisions. The counselors listen to and encourage individuals to talk about their situation and their feelings, and empathize, that is, they show that they understand how the person is feeling. The counselors give them accurate, clear information to help them to make decisions and try to give them support and confidence to do what they decide.

UNAIDS defines counseling as "a confidential dialogue between a client and a counselor aimed at enabling the client to cope with stress and take personal decisions related to HIV/AIDS."

Counseling is different from advising. When you advise others you tell them what you think they should do. When you counsel you do not impose your own ideas and values.

In many societies counseling may be a new and unfamiliar idea. When people have problems they traditionally take them to an older family member who is likely to tell them what to do. However, people from any culture are usually glad to have the opportunity to talk about their worries with someone who will listen, is well informed, will not judge them, and will not tell anyone else.

When can counseling be useful?

Some of the situations in which counseling can be helpful include:

- Someone who is considering having an HIV test or who has signs and symptoms of HIV infection may need *pre-test counseling*.

- Someone who receives an HIV test result may need *post-test counseling*.

- Post-abortion care, prenatal care, family planning care, treatment for sexually transmitted infections, and premarital counseling all provide opportunities for *prevention* or *behavior change counseling*.

- When individuals have problems they may benefit from *supportive and decision-making counseling*.

- Someone who has suffered a serious loss may benefit from *grief counseling*.

- Someone who is distressed may need *crisis counseling*.

The needs of people confronted with HIV change over time; counseling sessions need to reflect these changes. Families or couples may attend counseling sessions together, as long as they all agree to "share confidentiality." Specific counseling may be needed for:

- parents and siblings of an HIV-infected child,

- women, men, or children who have been sexually assaulted or abused,

- HIV-positive pregnant women,

- people who are dying and their families.

Training in counseling skills is an important component of several strategies and interventions, including voluntary counseling and testing (VCT) services (page 87), strengthening reproductive health services (page 148), behavior change for young people (page 100), establishing a continuum of care for those infected and affected (page 175), VCT during pregnancy (page 141), and counseling in relation to HIV and infant feeding (page 143).

What qualities does a counselor need to have?

Counselors need to be:

- good listeners,
- warm and caring,
- respected,
- well informed,
- motivated,
- resilient, and
- familiar with the cultural context and the history of displacement of the people they will counsel.

Different categories of workers can be trained in counseling skills. In humanitarian settings these workers might include:

- primary health care workers,
- social welfare workers,
- workers in sexual and gender-based violence programs,
- traditional birth attendants,
- family planning workers,
- teachers,
- people living with HIV,
- community volunteers, and
- ministers.

These skills are useful for communicating with and caring for all their clients, not only those with HIV infection. Some of these workers may already have counseling skills and experience but need to become well informed about HIV-related issues. They may be able to train others.

What sort of place is suitable for counseling?

Counseling can take place in many settings in clinics or hospitals or within the community. It is important to provide a setting that is private, comfortable, quiet, accessible, and able to protect confidentiality. In busy clinics it may not be possible for a room to be set aside for counseling, but with thought it may be possible to create a private space using curtains or screens. If a room or space is set aside, it is important not to label it as an HIV counseling room. If this room is within an MCH clinic men may feel awkward about attending.

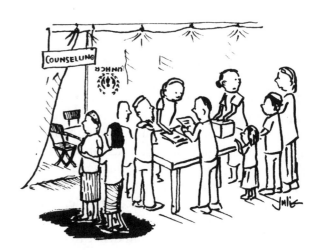

It is also important to ask whether different ethnic groups will be able to access the counseling site, especially marginalized groups who may be particularly vulnerable. All clinic staff need to understand the importance of a friendly and nondiscriminatory manner and the need for confidentiality.

Consider other possible sites for counseling in the camps or community. Consult with women, men, young people, elderly people, and different ethnic groups. They may each have different reasons for finding access difficult. It may be embarrassing or stigmatizing to visit a site that is used only for counseling, while a room within a youth center or administrative building may be noisy but more anonymous. Will the host population be able to access the site? If not, do they have access to alternative counseling services?

RATIONALE

Studies show that counseling can help people infected with HIV, and their families, to cope. Counseling can also help people to change behavior to avoid infection with HIV. But counseling cannot be effective unless it is properly supported, coordinated, and funded. Training too few counselors and expecting them to work on their own can be harmful for the clients and the counselors. Service managers and policy makers need to be convinced that counseling is valuable, and they need to understand that counselors require training and supervision. It may be important for NGO staff to play an advocacy role. Be able to explain simply what counseling is and the role it can play.

A number of studies and evaluations have been carried out. Try to identify studies that are locally relevant to use for advocacy with local officials.

A randomized controlled study of voluntary counseling and testing compared to basic health information in sites in Tanzania, Kenya, and Trinidad found that the proportion of individuals reporting unprotected intercourse decreased more in the group who received voluntary counseling and testing than in the group who received health information alone.[1]

In Uganda, The AIDS Support Organisation (TASO) conducted a study on 730 HIV-positive clients to whom it had given long-term counseling. Counseling appeared to help these clients cope with their infection. Of the clients sampled, 90 percent had revealed the fact of their infection to another person, with 85.3 percent telling relations. TASO clients who had received regular counseling also reported a high level of acceptance of HIV-positive people within families and in communities.[2]

Community-based counseling for behavioral change has been successfully provided in a rural Medical Research Council project in western Uganda, where condom use increased from two thousand to seven thousand per month.[3]

In 1992, a study in Rwanda examined the impact of preventive counseling. It was shown that for the women whose partners were also counseled and tested the annual incidence of new HIV infections decreased from 4.1 percent to 1.8 percent. Among women who were HIV-positive, the prevalence of gonorrhea decreased from 13 percent to 6 percent, with the greatest reduction in those using condoms.[4]

It is difficult to measure the effects of counseling interventions. If you are able to, it is valuable to document the process of implementing counseling strategies and evaluate the impact. Be sure to publish your experiences through journal or newsletter articles.

STRATEGIES

- Train counselors.
- Prepare checklists.
- Support counselors.
- Publicize availability of counseling (see page 100).

Training of counselors

It is not necessary to train as a psychologist to be a counselor. However, it is not enough simply to have a caring personality. Counseling requires training in specific skills that include:

- listening in an open and nonjudgmental way,
- asking supportive questions,
- discussing options,
- encouraging the client to make his or her own informed decisions,
- giving accurate information, and
- arranging follow-up.

A short period of training in counseling can improve the skills and confidence of health care and social workers. After the initial training counselors should receive support and supervision in their work and participate in a further training workshop several months later.

It is important to select trainee counselors carefully; they should be people who will be

1. The Voluntary HIV-1 Counseling and Testing Efficacy Study Group, "Efficacy of Voluntary HIV-1 Counseling and Testing in Individuals and Couples in Kenya, Tanzania, and Trinidad: A Randomized Trial," *Lancet* 356 (2000): 103–12.

2. TASO, *Uganda — the Inside Story: Participatory Evaluation of HIV/AIDS Counseling, Medical, and Social Services, 1993–94* (Kampala: TASO, 1995). WHO/GPA/TCO/HCS/95.1.

3. F. Mugula et al., "A Community-based Counseling Service as a Potential Outlet for Condom Distribution," Ninth International Conference on AIDS and STD in Africa, Kampala, December 1995 (paper WeD834).

4. S. Allen et al., "Confidential HIV Testing and Condom Promotion in Africa: Impact on HIV and Gonorrhoea Rates," *Journal of the American Medical Association* 268 (1992): 3338–43.

in a position to counsel others as part of their job. TASO (Uganda) suggests a useful approach to trainee selection. They conduct a one-day AIDS counseling awareness workshop for a large group of people being considered for training. During the workshop they raise controversial issues such as compulsory partner notification. The trainers observe the attitudes, reactions, and interpersonal interaction skills of the prospective trainees and, based on this, select people for the counseling skills training.

During the training it is most important to include a session discussing the meaning and practice of confidentiality. Refugees and IDPs may have reasons to feel very insecure and to fear serious consequences if other people learn about their status. Counselors need to have a clear understanding of why confidentiality is so important, and that it is important not just to practice it, but to tell clients that everything that is said will remain confidential and that their HIV status will not be disclosed without their consent. Confidentiality may be difficult to maintain in overcrowded clinics. When chatting with friends after work it can be very tempting to mention something about a client that the counselor has learned within a counseling session. How to safeguard confidentiality when documenting counseling sessions or referring clients to other services are challenges that need to be resolved through discussion. Trainees should be encouraged to discuss solutions for their particular setting. In some circumstances it may be best not to record any personal information about clients. If the counselor writes on a client-held health card it is important to be sure that the client knows what has been written.

It is also important for the trainees to understand denial. Denial may be a powerful and unconscious influence on behavior. Denial can prevent people from seeking treatment, accepting an HIV test, and coming back for results of a test if they have one. Denial can prevent people from telling their sexual partner about their infection or practicing safe sex to protect others, and may result in aggressive reactions toward counselors and partners who raise these issues.

Information for trainees about counseling in different situations

This information is aimed at the trainee counselors, and could be adapted or translated and used as handouts.

Pre-test counseling

Why is it necessary to counsel before doing an HIV antibody test?

Pre-test counseling is necessary to enable the individuals to reach an informed decision about whether to have the test or not and, if they decide to have it, to prepare them for the result.

Why is it necessary for the client to make an informed decision?

There is no cure for HIV infection as there is for syphilis or gonorrhea. There may be disadvantages to having the test, and it is important for the client to consider the disadvantages and advantages before deciding.

A client who has been prepared may be less disturbed by a positive result. When individuals receive a positive test result, they are often too shocked or upset to take in what they need to know about HIV, so it is important to give information before the test.

In pre-test counseling the counselor explores with the individuals behavior that may have placed them at risk. Testing for HIV, when accompanied by pre-test counseling, is a very important component of prevention of spread of HIV. The persons realize that the possibility that they may be infected with HIV is real and that they need to change their behavior whether the test result is positive or negative.

In refugee/IDP or refugee-impacted settings it is important to bear in mind what may have happened to the clients during the conflict or emergency that led to their displacement and the changed social context in which they now live. Many displaced women will have experienced rape or coercive sex, or may have been obliged to have sex in exchange for food for their family. They may have lost their partner and other family members. They may have special reason to fear having an HIV test and may become upset when asked about whether they have been at risk. They may still be experiencing risk that they are not able to control.

⚭ DISCUSSION POINT ⚭

Some people worry that the principles of confidentiality and informed consent lead to more spread of HIV. They worry particularly that the wives of infected men are exposed to risk when their husbands do not know their status, or will not tell their wives and use condoms. Experience from many countries shows that these principles do not increase the spread of HIV, but can increase the likelihood that people will come forward for counseling and testing. Denial, stigma, and discrimination result in secrecy and are obstacles to an effective response to HIV. What are the best ways to reduce denial, stigma, and discrimination and to open up the epidemic?

UNAIDS and WHO offer suggestions in the document *Opening Up the HIV Epidemic: Guidance on Encouraging Beneficial Disclosure, Ethical Partner Counseling, and Appropriate Use of HIV Case Reporting.* November 2000. Available from UNAIDS or at *www.unaids.org.*

—*Questions and Answers on Reporting, Partner Notification and Disclosure of HIV Serostatus and/or AIDS, Public Health and Human Rights Implications.* Geneva: WHO/UNAIDS, June 1999 (UNAIDS/00.26E).

Men and children may also have experienced sexual assault. In the context of pre-test counseling it needs to be clear to both counselor and client what the agenda of the session is — "We are here to discuss the possibility of an HIV test." If difficult issues do come up counselors can listen and empathize but should not feel that they must address the issue themselves. They may decide that an HIV test would not be appropriate at that time and if possible refer the client.

Many women find it easier to discuss the possibility of HIV infection with their partner than to tell him that they have had a positive test. Ask the woman if she would prefer to talk to her partner or bring him for counseling before you test her blood. Then, if both agree, you can test their blood at the same time. When both partners are infected, sometimes one blames the other. It can be helpful to discuss this possibility with the couple, and explain why such blaming is inappropriate, before the tests.

During pre-test counseling it is important to discuss who the client might tell if the result is positive. In humanitarian settings there is often a very high level of concern about confidentiality. Explain clearly how the results will be handled and how confidentiality will be maintained. When people are open about their HIV infection, it is easier for them to receive help and support. Others may decide to protect themselves against infection, and stigma may become less in a community where many are open about their infection. Keeping the diagnosis secret is stressful. For these reasons it is reasonable to encourage (but not to force) disclosure. There are different levels of disclosure. Some might want to tell only their partner. Others might be comfortable telling their closest family members or friends, or they might be willing to be publicly open about their HIV status. At the pre-test counseling session you might discuss the first two levels of disclosure — but it is more appropriate to delay discussion about being publicly open until later.

What are the possible advantages and disadvantages of having an HIV test that you should be prepared to discuss with a client? Remember that the advantages and disadvantages vary with individuals and with their

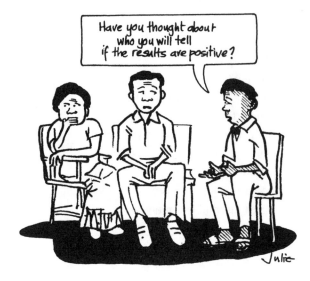

circumstances. Helping clients to see which is important for them is a counseling skill.

Possible *advantages* include:

- Having the test may reduce the anxiety of not knowing whether they are infected.

- They will be in a better position to make decisions about the future (such as whether to become pregnant or not).

- If they are infected, opportunistic infections can be treated more quickly, and unnecessary tests avoided.

- If they are infected, they may be motivated to take up a healthier lifestyle.

- There may be benefits that they become entitled to if they are known to be HIV positive.

Possible *disadvantages* include:

- If others learn that they are HIV positive, the clients may be stigmatized.

- They may be rejected by partner or family.

- Women may lose financial support if their husband learns that they had a positive test result.

- Travel to other countries may be limited.

- They may be unable to obtain life insurance or a mortgage.

Why do people find AIDS a difficult disease to understand?

Many people do not know about the immune system. People often find it difficult to understand why different AIDS patients suffer from such different symptoms. It can be helpful to describe the immune system as the "defense army" of the body. HIV attacks the "soldiers" (white cells). It is easy to understand that disease of the sex organs can be spread sexually. But many find it hard to believe that HIV, which causes symptoms in other parts of the body, can be transmitted sexually. The fact that someone who is well can be infectious also causes confusion.

The following tips can help clients to remember information:

- Be brief. Try not to give too much information. Emphasize the important points.

- Organize the information. Explain to the client how you organize the information.

- Give the most important information first.

- Be simple. Use short sentences and simple words. Avoid technical terms.

- Repeat the most important information.

- Be specific. Say, "You can get condoms free from the Family Planning Clinic near the market," not "Condoms are easy to get."

- Give information slowly.

- Ask clients to repeat back to you in their own words what you have said.

Post-test counseling

When individuals arrive to obtain their result try not to keep them waiting for a long time. Once they are sitting down, tell them the result in a straightforward way. Give them time to respond before giving them any information. Give individuals their test results only when there is enough time to counsel them.

Common reaction stages that many people pass through when they learn that they are HIV antibody positive include shock, fear, anxiety, denial, anger, blame, resignation or depression, and acceptance. One of the aims of post-test counseling is to help persons to pass through these stages to reach an acceptance of their condition. This is likely to take more than one session, and some people may need several further sessions.

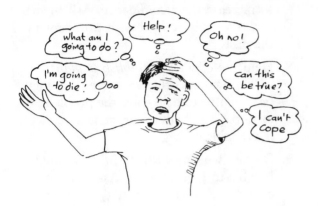

People may express their initial distress in different ways.

- Some cry. This is a natural response. Give them time to cry.

- Persons who are shocked may appear to listen to you but do not take in anything that you say. They may fall quiet for a long time. You need to ask questions that may engage them.

- Some express anger. It is important that you do not take offense.

- Some become agitated. You must remain calm yourself.

The content of a post-test counseling session will vary with different individuals. It depends on the emotional state of the clients, their level of understanding, their cultural beliefs, and whether they already have HIV-related illness. It can be helpful to talk about the idea of living positively with HIV. Emphasize that being infected with HIV is not the same as having AIDS, and that they may have many years of healthy life ahead.

In humanitarian settings people who test positive for HIV are likely to be very concerned about the consequences if people find out. Reassure them that you will not tell anyone.

The need for a "crisis counseling" approach can arise during post-test counseling. When persons feel overwhelmed by a problem, they become distressed or agitated. They feel that they have lost control and do not know what to do. The aim of "crisis counseling" is to restore a sense of control (see page 75).

Many people find it difficult to tell their spouse or sex partner about a positive result. Ask them how they think that their partner will react. If appropriate, ask them how they have coped when their partner has reacted like this in the past. Clients may find it helpful to role-play with the counselor how they will tell their partner. The counselor might offer to be present when the client tells his or her partner.

You may be tempted to falsely reassure clients — for example, to say that they will not become ill. This is not helpful, because when they do become ill, they will lose confidence in you. Also, it encourages both client and counselor to avoid facing difficult issues such as dying.

Clients often forget what was said after they receive a positive result. Give literate clients a leaflet with the most important facts simply explained for them to read later. Many clients will benefit from a second counseling session one week later when they have had a chance to think about the implications of their diagnosis and have more questions. A few clients will need several sessions. In humanitarian settings there are likely to be few counselors. If there is a local support group, refer the client. But if you determine that the client has little social support, offer a follow-up visit.

Post-test counseling is also necessary when the test result is negative. A negative result can make a person feel free to continue high-risk behavior, so you need to repeat advice about preventing the spread of HIV. If the person was infected recently and has not yet produced antibodies, the result may be a false negative (the window period). If the patient has been at risk, suggest another test in three months.

Supportive and problem-solving counseling

After the shock of learning that they have HIV has passed, people with HIV face many problems. They may find it helpful to be able to talk to a counselor about their concerns — it does not have to be the same counselor. The aim of problem-solving counseling is to help them to reach and carry out decisions to enable them to cope with their problems. These might include:

- decisions to change high-risk behavior, or to talk to their partner about high-risk behavior,

- decisions about who to tell about the diagnosis, and when and how to tell them,

- decisions about how to care for children or other dependents,

- decisions about whether to have more children.

Problem-solving counseling includes the following steps:

1. *Listen* carefully. Allow clients to describe their problems in their own way. Encourage them to express their feelings and fears: "What frightens you most when you think about telling your wife/husband?"

2. *Show empathy*, which means showing that you know how they feel, and support. For example: "That must worry you a lot," "Did you find that frustrating?" "It is not surprising that you feel anxious/angry/depressed. I am here and can help you with this problem."

3. *Summarize* what the client has said. This clarifies exactly what the problem is and lets the client know that you have heard. Ask whether you have understood the problem correctly.

4. Help clients to *prioritize* their problems. They may feel overwhelmed: "It's so awful, I can't begin to think what to do." It can help to identify which problems they feel are most important: "What is your greatest worry?" ("That I will be dependent on others") "What worries you most about being dependent?" and so on.

5. *Clarify the possible alternative courses of action*. Make suggestions (without telling the client what to do): "Have you thought of . . . " or "What might happen if. . . . " If you explore the consequences of taking different courses of action, you can help clients to reach a decision. Summarize the options.

6. *Provide any factual information* that they need on which to base decisions.

7. *Help clients to put their decisions into practice*. Discuss their strengths and skills to increase their confidence. Ask them how they have coped with problems in the past.

8. Help the client to *establish a plan of action*. Discuss other resources that might be available to help solve the problem, for example, legal advice or welfare services, if available.

9. Discuss which *family and friends* might be able to give support. Ask about the client's religious or spiritual beliefs.

10. Put them in touch with local *support* groups.

Some clients may deny their HIV status. Sometimes what may seem like denial is a genuine lack of understanding. For others denial is a way to cope with an unacceptable truth. Do not force these patients to face reality because they may react with explosive emotions, becoming very anxious or aggressive. The counselor needs to adopt a gradual and sensitive approach.

Displaced and conflict-affected populations may have so many other problems to cope with that the idea that in years to come they will become sick and die of AIDS may not seem like a priority. They may be more worried about their short-term survival.

The counselor cannot take responsibility for providing for all the clients' needs but should be able to refer them to other services that might be available. It can be tempting to try to solve the clients' problems for them. This can lead to dependence. If you arrange counseling sessions too frequently, clients may begin to feel that they cannot do without you.

Counselors need to be aware that neurological and psychiatric complications of HIV infection may affect a client's behavior.

Fears of dying, of serious illness, or of a partner leaving may be difficult to talk about. But they are easier to talk about before a patient becomes seriously ill. Do not avoid talking about these fears, although people may fear that talking about death will bring bad luck.

People who have accepted that they have AIDS will be able to prepare for dying. They may have family problems that they would like to resolve; they may need to arrange for care of their children and prepare a will. They need to be able to choose whether to die at home or in the hospital; they need acceptance from staff, family, and friends so that they can die with dignity. They also need relief from pain and discomfort (see page 178).

The counselor can help a client to prepare instructions in the form of a will. This can:

- bring peace of mind to people who know they are dying,

- prevent their assets being lost by their spouse or children,

- ensure that they are able to choose a suitable guardian for their children,

- reduce the chance of legal fights after the death,

- lessen worries about insecurity,

- state how and where they wish to be buried or cremated.

Crisis counseling

A crisis may be precipitated by a variety of problems: some may have been told that they have HIV, or find that their spouse or child is infected; others may fear that they have been exposed, for example, through a needle-stick injury. In a crisis, people feel helpless and anxious. They may suddenly feel intensely threatened and appear to react irrationally. Counselors who remain calm can help agitated clients to calm themselves.

1. First ensure the safety of the clients and others, including yourself.

2. Take steps to help clients calm down: ask them to sit down, get them a sweet warm drink.

3. Do not offer false reassurance, or give advice, or take offense.

4. Offer acceptance and support: "You are very anxious. You need to talk about this. I have time to listen to you."

5. When the client is calmer, ask questions to find out more about the problem and the patient's circumstances.

6. Ask about the client's present feelings and fears. (This is not an appropriate time to ask about the client's past). Summarize your understanding of the problem.

7. Find out what the client thinks is the worst aspect of the crisis.

8. Discuss what needs to be done most urgently to contain the crisis now.

9. Agree on a small task that the client can carry out, with support. For example, individuals may feel that they can never return to work because they think fellow workers have discovered that they have HIV. An appropriate small task might be for them to visit a fellow worker for a chat. Performing such a task can help to ease the crisis and restore a sense of control.

10. Arrange a further session to discuss longer-term solutions to the problem.

Prevention counseling

Prevention counseling is similar to one-to-one health education. However, counseling is a deeper, more personal, and more detailed process. The counselor provides information and encourages patients to discuss their feelings and attitudes, and together they explore obstacles to behavior change. If a health care worker simply tells patients what they should do, it may increase their resistance to changing their behavior.

The principles of counseling for prevention have been described already. The key is engaging clients to think about the ways that they may be vulnerable to infection with HIV. Remember that some people have little control over the factors that put them at risk of infection with HIV. Be wary of suggesting simple solutions.

Counseling for children

The HIV epidemic often places great responsibilities and stresses on children. Counseling may help them to cope when their parents are ill or dying, or with worries about their own infection. They may face discrimination because of HIV in the family. The siblings of infected children also often need attention and support. Older children may need counseling related to sexual issues. Children may have been sexually abused and need supportive counseling in relation to this.

Role-play training exercise

Role-play is especially helpful in counseling training, as participants have the opportunity to practice skills and gain confidence in a safe situation. Below there are some scenarios that may arise in relation to HIV infection. The names may be changed to locally familiar ones, and the scenarios copied onto cards. More scenarios appropriate to the context may need to be prepared.

The participants work in groups of three or four. Each group takes a card. One participant plays the client, and another plays the counselor. The others observe what is helpful and what is not. After the role-play has finished they are asked to give positive comments first and then make some suggestions for improvements. Then the group takes another card, and they change roles. All the small groups may perform the same role-play situation and discuss all the observations together afterward.

In real life, a counseling session may last from fifteen minutes to one hour. In this exercise it will be necessary to limit the time for each role-play to about fifteen minutes. Participants should be reassured that they are not expected to "complete" the counseling "sessions" in that time. It can be helpful to identify a specific task for the trainees to practice. For example, for Ned's scenario the task could be to find out what he knows about HIV and correct misconceptions. In Angela's role-play the task could be to discuss home-based care options.

To be sure that the exercise is successful it needs to be led by someone with experience of counseling. If participants try the exercise without enough help, they may find that they do not know what to do, which may reduce their confidence in their ability to counsel clients in real life. Ideally, the facilitator should give a demonstration of role-playing counseling with another

leader or with a participant before participants attempt it themselves. Then, while the groups work, the facilitator circulates to comment and to sort out any problems that arise. It may be helpful to have the checklists available to the participants.

The facilitator needs to pay attention to the information and suggestions that the "counselor" gives to the "client." Information must be accurate and appropriate for the situation, and corrected if necessary. The facilitator also needs to pay attention to the way in which the "counselor" handles the "client." They should listen, empathize, explore possible solutions to problems, help with decisions, and give support. They must communicate well. They should not impose their own ideas and values. Many health workers find this difficult at first, because in their training they have often learned to give patients clear advice.

Role-play can be a powerful training tool. Participants temporarily adopt the character of the role they are playing and may experience the corresponding emotions. At the end it is important to have an informal discussion in order to debrief and restore the participants to their own roles.

Pre-test counseling scenarios

Rose is an eighteen-year-old girl who has been in the camp for six months. She has been referred for pre-test counseling because she presented with an STI. On the long walk to the camp she was raped by two soldiers. She has to fetch wood each day and has been raped several times since she arrived at the camp.

Ned is a young man in the camp hospital with severe pulmonary tuberculosis. His doctor has referred him to you for pre-test counseling.

Mary, aged twenty-five, was displaced from her home with all her neighbors, two years ago. She was raped repeatedly by soldiers at that time. She has heard about AIDS and has come to talk about having a test for HIV. Mary is single.

Post-test counseling scenarios

Jenny is twenty, single, with no children. She works in a bar in the refugee/IDP camp. She had herpes zoster, but is now well. She has come to the clinic for the result of her HIV antibody test, which is positive.

Angela is a thirty-five-year-old nurse's aide, married with five children. She had been losing weight and feeling weak. She now comes to you to hear the result of her HIV antibody test, which is positive.

Peter, aged eighteen, was referred for counseling and testing because he had an STI. The HIV test result is negative.

Anna and her husband, Bernard, have one child aged eighteen months, who has HIV infection and who gets ill frequently. They have been thinking recently about having another child.

Charles is a twenty-two-year-old student. He has known that he is infected with HIV for ten months. His health is good and he has accepted his condition. He comes to you now because he has a new girlfriend and he wants to find out where he can get condoms.

Marie is thirty years old and has three small children. In recent months she has lost a lot of weight and has had recurrent illnesses. She feels sure that she has AIDS. She is troubled because although she is fond of her husband and he has cared for her during her illnesses, she feels very angry with him for infecting her with this fatal virus, which he will not admit.

Stella, aged twenty-four, is ill with HIV infection. She knows that she is infected and she has been counseled. She is now well enough to go home, but asks to see the counselor again because she cannot decide whether to tell her husband. Stella was divorced before she met her present husband, who has a second older wife.

Crisis counseling scenarios

Mathias is forty-two, married with seven children. He arrives at the outpatient clinic in a very aggressive and angry mood. His wife has just come home and told him that she is infected with HIV. He blames the health worker for testing his wife without his consent.

Joseph, a teacher aged twenty-five, has come to you in an extremely agitated state. At a pre-migration medical examination a doctor found some enlarged glands and suggested that he have an HIV antibody test. He is referred to you for counseling.

Prevention counseling scenarios

Anne, aged twenty-three, was admitted with bleeding following an illegal abortion. All women who have had an abortion are offered a chance to talk with the counselor. What will you say to her?

Simon, aged eighteen, has attended the clinic for treatment of a severe chancroid ulcer. He needs prevention counseling as well as antibiotics.

Bereavement counseling scenarios

John's wife died two weeks ago of an AIDS-related illness. Their baby girl died six months ago at the age of two. John has been left with a four-year-old boy. John's brother has brought him to the counselor because he has been sitting in his hut and not looking after his son. John has not had an HIV test.

Sarah is an elderly widow. Her youngest son died of AIDS, aged twenty, one month ago. Her second son died in the recent armed conflict, and two of her daughters died of AIDS in the past five years. A neighbor suggested she come for counseling because she is not sleeping or eating well and cries frequently.

Preparation of checklists

It is helpful to inexperienced counselors to have printed checklists to consult when counseling. The checklists we provide at the end of this chapter will need to be modified to make them locally appropriate. Participants could undertake this task and then use the checklists in role-play practice. After this the checklists should be tested by both experienced and inexperienced counselors and modified before printing. The checklists will last longer if they are laminated or put in a clear plastic envelope.

It is helpful to prepare a checklist of points that you want to cover. Tell the trainees to keep the checklists with them when they counsel until they become experienced. Tell them not to be embarrassed to look at the checklist when they are counseling. They can say, "There is a lot to explain—I want to make sure that I do not miss anything."

Support for counselors

Although there can be a great deal of satisfaction in providing support to people through counseling it can also be very stressful. Counselors can become emotionally exhausted or "burnt out." They feel tired and become irritable or depressed. It is essential to provide counselors with an opportunity to talk in confidence about the challenges their clients present, preferably at regular meetings with a familiar supervisor. They may also wish to meet in a group informally to share their experiences.

Counselors often have a position as a nurse or a social worker, and their supervisors may expect them to give priority to tasks other than counseling. Counselors may then visit their clients on a voluntary basis and become exhausted. Administrative support can reduce stress by providing appropriate timetables, with rotation of tasks, clear job descriptions, and reasonable working facilities. It is important for managers and supervisors of counselors to identify mechanisms to reward commitment and maintain motivation. These might include awards, opportunities to attend conferences, and the chance to assist in training new counselors.

Counselors often feel frustrated because they have few ways to help their client — for example, when they counsel women who are exposed to the risk of HIV but are unable to do anything about it. Supervisors might arrange for them to talk in confidence (with the woman's permission) with appropriate officials, social welfare workers, or sexual and gender-based violence program workers to determine an appropriate plan to protect the woman. Counselors need to be able to work closely with others to lessen feelings of isolation and powerlessness. Supervisors may need to help counselors to see that there are inevitably limits to the help that they can give and to prevent them from feeling responsible for factors that are beyond their control.

The resources needed to provide these supports for counselors should be considered a necessary part of the counseling program budget and an investment, since if necessary supports are ignored the turnover of counselors will be high.

ADDITIONAL RESOURCES

James-Traore, Tijuana A., and Valerie Flax. *Counselor Training: A Manual for Counseling Adolescents with a Special Emphasis on Reproductive Health.* New York: IRC, March 1998.

Meursing, K., and F. Sibindi. "HIV Counseling — A Luxury or a Necessity?" *Health Policy and Planning* 15 (2000): 17–23.

TASO. *HIV/AIDS Counseling: The TASO Experience* (1998). A thirty-minute video illustrating TASO's approach to counseling. Available in French, English, and Swahili. Available from TALC (free for organizations in sub-Saharan Africa).

WHO/GPA. *Counseling for HIV/AIDS: A Key to Caring.* Geneva: WHO, 1995. WHO/GPA/TCO/HCS/95.15. For policy makers, planners, and implementers of counseling activities. Explores programmatic and policy issues with regard to planning and setting up counseling services.

WHO/GPA. *Source Book for HIV/AIDS Counseling Training.* WHO, 1994. WHO/GPA/TCO/HCS/94.9. For training counselors. Deals with initial training and refresher courses.

WHO/UNAIDS. *Questions and Answers on Reporting, Partner Notification, and Disclosure of HIV Serostatus and/or AIDS: Public Health and Human Rights Implications.* Geneva, WHO/UNAIDS, June 1999.

Internet resources

"UNAIDS Technical Update: Counseling and HIV/AIDS." November 1997. Available at *www.unaids.org.*

CHECKLIST FOR PRE-TEST COUNSELING

- Introduce yourself.
- Explain that the interview is completely confidential.
- Explain why the doctor or nurse has suggested an HIV antibody test, or explore why the client is requesting the test.
- Assess with clients behaviors that may have exposed them to infection with the virus.
- Ask what clients already know about HIV transmission and prevention.
- Correct any false beliefs and explain the basic facts about HIV infection and how it is spread:
  - how HIV affects the immune system
  - how HIV differs from AIDS
  - that there is a long incubation period
  - how HIV is transmitted
  - how HIV does not spread
  - that there is no cure at present
  - that treatment for opportunistic infections is available
  - that treatment for symptoms is available
  - that there is hope that there may be a cure in future
- Explain that the HIV antibody test is not a test for AIDS.
- Explain the "window period," that is, the time between infection and the development of antibodies (seroconversion), when the test is negative but the person is infected and infectious.
- Explain how long it takes for the test results to be available and discuss how the client will cope during the waiting time.
- Explain policies for confirmatory tests and for follow-up.
- Ask about family circumstances and identify what support they have from family and friends.
- Discuss the personal implications of a positive result: Whom would they tell? How might they cope with a positive result? Explore the advantages of disclosure.
- Discuss some of the practical issues, e.g., how to use and where to get condoms and family planning advice.
- If clients keep their own health care record, tell them what you write on it so that they can protect their confidentiality.
- Check the client's understanding.
- Arrange a follow-up appointment.

CHECKLIST FOR POST-TEST COUNSELING
WHEN THE TEST IS NEGATIVE

- Greet the clients and tell them the result of the test.

- Check what they understand by the result.

- Explore whether they have been at risk in the past three months. If so, explain that they may be infected and should have another test in three month's time.

- Explain the importance of maintaining safe behavior. Ask them what difficulties they might have in avoiding risky behaviors.

  - If relevant, show them a condom and explain how to use condoms properly.

  - Let them know that if they have difficulties they can return for further counseling.

- Ask them to tell their peers about the risk of HIV infection and how to protect themselves.

CHECKLIST FOR POST-TEST COUNSELING
WHEN THE TEST IS POSITIVE

- Greet the clients and tell them the result of the test.

- Give them time to react.

- Check that they understand the meaning of the test result and the difference between HIV infection and AIDS.

- Ask them what worries them most about the result; discuss alternatives for dealing with this worry.

- Check their knowledge of HIV and its transmission.

- Explain any facts that they have forgotten or misunderstood.

- Ask if they will find it difficult to tell their sex partner/s.

    - Help them to plan how to do this.

    - Invite them to bring their partner for counseling.

- Ask them who else they plan to tell. Identify what emotional support they have from family and friends.

- Discuss the responsibility to protect others. Ask about risk behavior, and discuss how they might change.

- Repeat information about "safer sex." If relevant, show them a condom and explain how to use condoms properly.

- Explain the practical precautions they need to take in the home.

- Give them time to ask questions.

- Put them in touch with local support groups.

- Explain the medical follow-up procedure. Stress that, although there is no cure, symptoms that might develop can be treated. Advise them to come early for treatment.

- Arrange a further appointment.

- Provide written information (if they are literate).

SUGGESTED INDICATORS

Indicator	*Method of measurement*
Checklists available in counseling settings	Observation
Number of counselors trained	Review of training course reports
Proportion of counselors assessed as competent after training	Assessment of competence of trainee through performance during role-play of counseling situations using a checklist
Proportion of women seen for post-abortion care who receive HIV counseling	Review of clinic records
Proportion of STI patients who receive counseling (by age and sex)	Review of clinic records
Level of community awareness of counseling services (both refugee/IDP and host) Ability of community to access counseling services Level of trust in confidentiality	Participatory appraisal and FGDs with community
Attendance at VCT services* (by age and sex)	Review of VCT service records
Satisfaction of clients with quality of counseling	Interviews with a sample of (consenting) clients—use checklist to see whether points have been covered. Ask about level of satisfaction with the counseling.
Satisfaction of counselors with level of support	Regular discussions with (1) counselors and (2) supervisors using a checklist

*Although it is interesting to follow trends over time in acceptance of HIV testing, it is not a good idea to use "Number of HIV tests" as an indicator of effective counseling. The purpose of pre-test counseling is to assist the person to reach his or her own decision about whether to have a test or not. Counselors should not feel that they are being evaluated by the number of clients that they "persuade" to have an HIV test.

8

Preventing Transmission through Sex

Sex is the most common route of transmission of HIV. Sexual activity, illness, and death are often taboo subjects, so promoting change to safer sexual practices is difficult. Safer sexual practices include:

- consistent use of condoms,
- nonpenetrative sex (e.g., mutual masturbation, sex between the thighs),
- sex with a single uninfected faithful partner,
- abstinence.

Impact of displacement on sexual practices and attitudes

Patterns of sexual behavior are likely to be altered by displacement. It is essential to analyze the changes and their probable impact. In a refugee/IDP camp with many single women and possibly poorly disciplined military groups in charge there are likely to be increased levels of violent or coercive sex. There may be mixing of groups with different rates of HIV. For example, a study in two Mozambican refugee/IDP camps in different parts of Swaziland found a much higher rate of HIV in the camp where there had been interaction between refugees/IDPs and the local population who had a high rate of HIV.[1] There may be soldiers from countries with a high prevalence of HIV deployed as international peacekeepers to an area with low rates of HIV. Single soldiers away from their wives and girlfriends are likely to pay for sex or start relationships with local women. This may be the starting point for a new epidemic of HIV in a vulnerable population. The usual restraints on young people may be lacking, and lack of activities and structure

result in boredom and a search for excitement. They may be more likely to have sex at an earlier age and with more partners. Where displaced people are living with host families, changes in sexual practices may be less significant, but overcrowding, enforced intimacy, and lack of privacy may affect sexual relationships. In countries where law and order no longer operate, women, young people, and children are often sexually exploited. They may be trafficked by organized criminals from one country to another and forced into prostitution.

Whatever the changes in sexual practices it is likely that the former societal attitudes and expectations will persist. This may prevent individuals from talking about their problems, and communities from recognizing and responding to the problems associated with changed sexual practices.

Attitudes toward pregnancy are also likely to be affected by displacement. Women may be fearful of becoming pregnant because of their uncertain future, their poverty, and the lack of services. If they have been raped, they may be distressed at the thought of becoming pregnant. On the other hand populations displaced as a result of armed conflict may want to see more babies being born and view promotion of family planning and condoms as attempts to prevent them from reproducing. This is an especially sensitive matter when ethnic groups have been targeted and expelled from their homes or killed in an attempt at genocide. These sensitivities need to be taken into account in planning condom promotion efforts.

The desire to see more babies born may mean that there is a general concern about infertility. Since the complications of STIs are the most common cause of infertility, the community's concern may be a powerful motivation toward adopting safer sexual practices. This might be

---

1. E. J. Van Rensburg, H. R. Lemmer, and J. J. Joubert, "Prevalence of Viral Infections in Mozambican Refugees in Swaziland," *East African Medical Journal* 72 (1995): 588–90.

used as a strong appeal in communication materials.

Although the most vulnerable groups for transmission through sex are generally the young and women, it is men who play the dominant role in deciding whether and under what circumstances sex will take place. It is therefore important to consider how to reach them with sexual behavior change programs.

Many HIV and STI programs have taken an approach that targets interventions narrowly to "high-risk groups," on the basis that if HIV can be prevented in these groups it will not reach the rest of the population. While it is important to identify and work with groups that are more vulnerable than others because they have a greater likelihood of unsafe sex encounters and lack access to services and information, there is need to be cautious. The groups most often targeted are sex workers, men who have sex with men, and truck drivers. When these groups are singled out for messages about reducing the numbers of their sexual partners and using condoms, they feel that they are being further marginalized and stigmatized. They suspect that the attention they receive is motivated by concern for the rest of the community rather than for themselves; this leads to resentment and rejection of messages. There is also a danger that as HIV becomes associated with these "high-risk" groups, other groups within the community may feel that they themselves are not at risk. The targeted interventions fail to reach people with the same behaviors as those in the "high-risk" groups who do not identify as "sex workers" or "men who have sex with men." In refugee/IDP settings a wide range of transactional sex may occur for different reasons. Soldiers may have sex with men but not identify themselves as homosexual or "gay." It is wise to explore appropriate ways to reach all the different groups in the community with relevant messages. Outreach and peer strategies tend to be the most effective with marginalized groups.

Behavior change strategies can succeed

Much has been learned in the past twenty years about preventing transmission of HIV through sex. Uganda and Thailand have been able to achieve large-scale changes in behavior that have resulted in decreased transmission of HIV; Senegal provides a valuable example of a poor country where HIV has not spread rapidly. It is difficult to be sure of the contribution of different factors to these successes. There are some features of the population that have been protective, but also evidence that actions carried out by communities, governments, and nongovernmental organizations have been effective. Some key features that seem to contribute to prevention of spread of HIV are:

* political leadership and openness about the threat of the epidemic;
* religious leadership;
* community leadership;
* sex education for young people and school children;
* outreach and peer programs for sex workers, their clients, and other vulnerable groups;
* STI control programs;
* promotion of condoms;
* access to testing for HIV in combination with counseling.

Thailand's 100 Percent Condom Program, for example, which aimed to make condom use universal among sex workers, has been one of the world's most successful condom promotion campaigns.

In Uganda among men aged fifteen to nineteen, the percentage who had ever used condoms rose from 20 percent in 1989 to about 60 percent in 1995 following a multi-sectoral program including condom distribution and promotion involving popular songs and drama groups, counseling, and support services. There is evidence that the reduction in prevalence of HIV in Uganda is also related to people having fewer sexual partners. Other factors that have been shown to slow the spread of HIV were knowing somebody who had died of AIDS, and talking with family and friends about the epidemic. Despite limited resources, Ugandans have developed personally and culturally appropriate behavioral strategies, which have dramatically reduced HIV prevalence.

Experience from Rwandan camps in Tanzania shows that such multi-sectoral approaches can be achieved in humanitarian settings.[2] A large-scale collaborative program was implemented in camps of more than 250,000 refugees. An initial community health survey of knowledge, attitudes, and practices provided baseline data. The program included distribution of free condoms and dissemination of HIV/AIDS information by community educators, treatment and counseling for STIs, mass education campaigns targeting adolescents and women as well as the general population, and creation of culturally specific videos in the local language to promote safer sexual behavior.

Some ideas about behavior change

To prevent the spread of HIV we need to change individual behaviors, such as having unprotected sex or sharing needles to inject drugs, although we recognize that individual behavior is part of a complex web of factors that influence risk of HIV in a community.

A talkback radio program asked its listeners how they were getting on with their New Year's resolutions. Some callers had tried to exercise more, some to give up fatty foods or smoking. Some had succeeded by stopping suddenly, others by cutting down gradually. Some had been helped by regular counseling, others by nonsmoking friends, and others by chewing nicotine gum. All had changed their behavior and they had done so using different strategies. But some useful lessons about effective behavior change strategies have been learned in recent years.

To make a resolution to change your behavior you need to have some sense that you can control your life. The examples of behavior change given above are likely to be meaningless to displaced and conflict-affected populations, who may have lost a sense of control, as well as their loved ones and their possessions. When they have to rely on donations to survive for long periods and have no opportunity to work

or determine their future, they suffer feelings of powerlessness and dependency. In these settings community-level strategies are likely to be more effective at reducing vulnerability to HIV and can create an environment that increases people's belief in their ability to take effective action.

Studies show that strategies that try to change individual behavior succeed only when people believe:

- they are susceptible to the problem;
- the problem is serious;
- their health will benefit if they change their behavior;
- the new behavior is socially desirable;
- the benefits will outweigh potential costs and barriers; and
- they have the ability to take effective action.[3]

People are more likely to change their behavior because of short-term consequences rather than more distant consequences. For example, a young man is more likely to use condoms to prevent a short-term consequence such as an STI or pregnancy than a longer-term consequence such as AIDS. What people view as socially desirable depends on what their peers think is socially desirable. A young man is more likely to use a condom if he feels that his friends think it's a normal and smart thing to do. In relation to sexual violence this theory suggests that we need to try to modify social norms to make sexual assault unacceptable and that it is important that penalties are strictly enforced so that there are short-term consequences to be feared from such behavior.

The Stages of Change Model[4] describes behavior change as a process, not an event.

- **Precontemplation:** The individuals have not begun to think about the need to change.
- **Contemplation:** Something happens to prompt them to start thinking about change.

---

2. J. A. Benjamin, E. Engel, and R. DeBuysscher, "AIDS Prevention Amid Chaos: The Case of Rwandan Refugees in Tanzania," International Conference on AIDS 11, no. 1 (July 1996): 225 (abstract no. Tu.D.24).

3. V. J. Strecher and I. M. Rosenstock, "The Health Belief Model," in K. Glanz et al., *Health Behavior and Health Education: Theory, Research and Practice* (San Francisco: Jossey-Bass, 1997).

4. J. O. Prochaska, C. C. DiClemente, and J. C. Norcross, "In Search of How People Change: Applications to Addictive Behaviors," *American Psychologist* 47 (1992): 1102–14.

- **Preparation:** They make a commitment to change. They might look for information and decide when they will change.

- **Action:** They begin to change their behavior.

- **Maintenance:** They sustain their behavior change and start to benefit. With practice the behavior becomes familiar and habitual.

The pace of progress through these stages is variable; people may become "stuck" at any stage. It can be helpful to counselors to have these stages in mind when they try to help people to achieve a change in behavior.

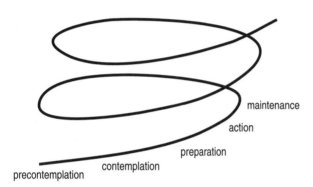

maintenance

action

preparation

precontemplation   contemplation

A Spiral of Behavior Change

—B. Parnell and K. Benton, *Facilitating Sustainable Behavior Change: A Guidebook for Designing HIV Programs* (Melbourne: Macfarlane Burnet Institute for Medical Research and Public Health, 1999).

Although individuals intend to maintain a new behavior, they might find it difficult. The resources they need, such as condoms, might cease to be available. People who supported the change might move away. For a range of reasons, people might move back to the earlier stages. But they never return to the precontemplation stage. Because people revert to an earlier pattern of behavior, this does not mean that they have "failed to change." Many people who eventually adopt a new habit make several attempts before the behavior is maintained long-term.

The enabling environment

Behavior does not occur in isolation; people respond to what is happening around them. The factors that influence positive change have

been described as making up an *enabling environment.*[5]

Social factors

An example of how the social and cultural context influences the prospects of behavior change relates to male homosexual behavior. In societies in which male homosexuality is taboo, men who want to have sex with men are more likely to marry but continue secretly to have sex with men. They may not admit even to themselves that they have sex with men. This makes it very difficult to reach this group with messages about safer sex behaviors. In this way social attitudes present a barrier to achieving behavior change, and these men and their wives remain vulnerable to infection with a fatal virus.

Religious factors

Religious beliefs are powerful influences on behavior. In some cultures religious prohibitions affect what can be discussed. If sex outside marriage is viewed as a sin, then it becomes difficult to discuss the issue, even though everyone may know that it is a common practice. Women may not feel that they can discuss their husband's infidelity or strategies to reduce the risk that results, even with other women.

Actions by leaders from many religions have contributed to HIV prevention and care. For this political and religious leadership to occur the leaders need information about the epidemic. As with other groups, peer education is effective. In many parts of the world religious groups have got together to form "faith-based networks" to share experiences about how best to contribute to both prevention and care. This can be important in shifting attitudes away from a judgmental and prohibitive approach. In Senegal, for example, conferences for senior Islamic leaders and Christian bishops led to an increase in support for people living with HIV, including acceptance of the use of condoms.

5. T. Kouda, "Responding to AIDS: Are There *Any* Appropriate Development and Health Policies?" *Journal of International Development* 7 (1995): 467–87.

The legal framework

Laws that prohibit certain behaviors can work against behavior change. For example, because using heroin or opium is illegal, people may inject rather than risk detection through the smell of smoking.

The extent to which laws are enforced is also important. In humanitarian settings there may be little chance that sexual assault or rape will be punished, even when evidence is available. There may be more than one system of law operating — and different groups enforcing their own rules to varying extents. The unpredictable nature of the enforcement of laws may make it a difficult environment in which to encourage behavior change. An unstable political environment may affect who can gain access to information and services necessary for behavior change. It is easier to obtain the cooperation of those responsible for law enforcement if they are included in planning strategies for behavior change.

Laws relating to freedom of access to information, discrimination, and advertising are also relevant.

Framework for planning interventions

At the end of part 2 we presented a framework for planning prevention interventions. Behavior change to prevent HIV depends upon services and supplies, including treatment for STIs, distribution of condoms, and access to voluntary counseling and testing for HIV. These are described in the next column under "Interventions that relate to provision of services." Advice for developing effective communication programs and other strategies to change individual behaviors is also presented. "Interventions that relate to the societal context" (page 110) presents some ideas for increasing the community's capacity to create an "enabling environment."

In this chapter we describe:

Interventions that relate to provision of services:

- Establish and promote VCT services.
- Promote and distribute condoms.
- Strengthen management and control of STIs.

Interventions that relate to changing individual behaviors:

- Develop and disseminate communication materials for behavior change.
- Promote peer education.
- Provide sex education for young people.
- Consider the role of HIV-positive people in prevention.
- Provide prevention counseling for STI patients.

Interventions that relate to the societal context:

- Prevent and manage the consequences of sexual and gender-based violence.
- Provide opportunities for social activities.
- Provide social activities for youth.
- Provide community communication activities to change attitudes.
- Support microfinance programs and income-generating activities.

The choice and design of these interventions will depend on the results of the local situation analysis.

INTERVENTIONS THAT RELATE TO PROVISION OF SERVICES

Establish and promote voluntary counseling and testing services

RATIONALE

Voluntary counseling and testing (VCT) services are part of a continuum of care and support for people with HIV. VCT can also be an effective prevention strategy, promoting behavior change among those who test negative as well as positive.[6]

Should you introduce VCT?

It is important to know whether refugees or IDPs had access to VCT in their home area, and whether VCT is available for the host population. In humanitarian settings VCT services

---

6. *Voluntary Counseling and Testing Technical Update,* UNAIDS, May 2000.

should be established only where there are relatively stable conditions and confidentiality can be guaranteed.

When you discuss whether you should introduce VCT ask yourselves:

1. Is there the technical capacity?

   - a regular, reliable, and sufficient supply of HIV test kits?

   - an appropriate testing strategy, including confirmatory testing of positive results as outlined in the *UNAIDS Policy on HIV Testing and Counseling* (see appendix B, page 199)?

   - high-quality testing and laboratory procedures in place to ensure accurate results?

   - systems in place to identify and correct technical and clerical errors?

2. Is there the staff capacity?

   - experienced health staff available who can take blood samples and who are trained to follow universal precautions?

   - trained counselors available to provide pre-test and post-test counseling?

   - support and supervision available for health workers and counselors?

   - laboratory staff trained in carrying out tests?

3. Is there the capacity for treatment and care?

   - medical treatment available for people diagnosed with HIV?

   - referral systems for the care and support of people who are diagnosed with HIV?

   - family and community support for people with HIV?

4. Is there the administrative capacity?

   - adequate space for confidential counseling and testing?

   - proper recording systems to ensure confidentiality and to make sure that people are given the correct results?

   - monitoring system for quality of counseling and testing services?

   - secure arrangements for supplies, transport, and storage?

5. Are there sufficient resources available?

   - to set up services, including training and improving laboratory infrastructure?

   - for recurrent costs such as purchases of tests and any additional staff salaries?

   - to run a comprehensive program that includes education, follow-up counseling, care, and support?

Informed consent

Informed consent requires an understanding of the implications of a positive test result and the voluntary decision to be tested. Pre-test counseling should include:

- the individuals' personal history and possible exposure to HIV,

- their personal context, including whether they have been exposed to violence, and

- their understanding of the modes of HIV transmission.

During post-test counseling, when the test result is positive, the person should be given emotional support and information about available care and social services (see page 73). If the HIV test is negative, then the person must be advised about the "window period" of three to six months when a negative result may be false. This counseling session is an important opportunity to discuss the way HIV spreads and methods of protection.

Mandatory testing violates human rights and does not contribute to public health. It is sometimes suggested:

- as a prerequisite to refugees' acceptance for resettlement to another country;

- as a part of pre-employment screening;

- as a prerequisite for surgery or other medical treatment;

- as part of premarital screening.

It is important to argue against mandatory testing in all these circumstances. Premarital testing for couples may be useful if the couple are counseled together and are tested voluntarily with informed consent.

If you establish VCT services, they need to be widely publicized. Increased awareness of VCT increases awareness of the risk of HIV. In publicity make clear that people can go to a VCT center for counseling even though they may not want an HIV test. They may be seeking answers to questions or advice about communicating with their partner about safe sex. It is also important that indicators for evaluating VCT centers measure trends in the numbers of people attending the center rather than the numbers tested.

Advantages and disadvantages of HIV testing

Advantages of testing include:

- improved health care, such as early treatment for tuberculosis and prevention of opportunistic infections with co-trimoxazole (see page 180);

- avoiding the expense of unnecessary screening tests and ineffective treatments;

- more informed decision making about the future;

- access to emotional and practical support;

- increased motivation to prevent HIV transmission;

- increased perception of vulnerability to HIV;

- alleviation of anxiety for those who test negative;

- more open and positive attitudes toward living with HIV, and reduced stigma;

- ability to make decisions about pregnancy and infant feeding.

The availability of VCT can create an environment in which more people are willing to be tested and helped to change their behavior, which in turn encourages beneficial disclosure.[7]

This is disclosure that is voluntary, respects the dignity of affected individuals, maintains confidentiality, and leads to greater openness about HIV in the community.

The disadvantages of testing include problems with coping with the result, and problems as a result of stigma, rejection, and discrimination. These were described in chapter 7. Other problems are the cost of testing and the possibility of inaccurate test results.

The planning team might conclude that while it is not feasible to implement a VCT service for all, it is possible to offer VCT to certain groups, such as pregnant women (see chapter 11), injecting drug users, sex workers and their clients, or patients with tuberculosis.

STRATEGIES

The steps to establish a VCT service are:

- Train counselors and supervisors (see chapter 7).

- Train laboratory staff in HIV testing.

- Establish systems for procurement, and secure storage of test kits.

- Establish system for confirmatory testing (see appendix B, page 199).

- Establish quality control for testing and laboratory procedures to ensure accurate and confidential results.

- Establish systems to minimize clerical errors.

- Identify and strengthen management, referral, and support options for those who test positive and their families.

- Promote and publicize VCT, especially to couples and youth.

- Establish a system for monitoring and evaluation.

Interpreting results of HIV antibody tests

Test results may be negative even though the individuals are infected if they are in the window period, that is, if they have not yet made enough antibodies for the test to detect. Test results may be positive even though the individuals are not infected. This is called a "false positive," and it is the reason why confirmatory tests are necessary before someone is given

---

7. UNAIDS, "Opening Up the HIV Epidemic: Guidance on Encouraging Beneficial Disclosure, Ethical Partner Counseling, and Use of HIV Case Reporting." November 2000. *www.unaids .org/publications/documents/epidemiology/surveillance/*.

FALSE POSITIVES

Assume that the false positive rate of the HIV antibody test is 0.5 percent.

Low prevalence population, e.g., 0.004 percent HIV infection rate.

Of 100,000 tests done, there will be 4 true positives and 500 false positives. The chance of any positive result being a false positive is 500/504 or 99 percent.

High prevalence population, e.g., 25 percent HIV infection rate.

Of 100,000 tests done, there will be 25,000 true positives and 500 false positives. The chance of any positive result being a false positive is 500/25,500, only 1.9 percent.

A real example is given by a study at the AIDS Reference Laboratory in Delhi in 1992. The staff found that when they tested blood donors (prevalence low at 0.1 percent), 31.7 percent of the positive results were false positives. However, when they tested thalassemic children who had had many transfusions (prevalence high at 8.5 percent), 100 percent of the positive results were confirmed as true positives.

a positive result. The chance that a positive test result is a false positive is greater in areas where HIV is rare. You can work through the example in the box above to see why this is.

Types of HIV tests

ELISA. The Enzyme Linked Immuno-Sorbent Assay (ELISA) HIV antibody test is most efficient for testing large numbers of samples each day. It is most commonly used for screening blood and for surveillance purposes. The testing kits require skilled technical staff, equipment, and a constant power supply, so they are not suitable for smaller or more isolated hospitals and clinics. The ELISA test is very sensitive, but a small percentage of false positive results do occur, so it is necessary to confirm positive results.

Rapid antibody tests. Several simple antibody tests (such as Serodia, Capillus, Multispot, HIV-CHEK, Determine) have been developed which are more suitable for use in small hospitals and laboratories. They are as sensitive and specific as ELISAs. Some take less than ten minutes to perform and so are called "rapid"

tests. They do not need trained technical staff or expensive equipment and are usually provided in kit form. Some of these tests are able to detect HIV antibodies in specimens of saliva or dried blood. There are four types: agglutination assays, comb/dipstick assays, flow-through membrane assays, and lateral flow membrane assays. In most of these, a positive result is indicated by the appearance of a clearly visible dot or line. Many of these tests have an internal sample addition control that validates each test run. The cost of an individual ELISA test is usually less than that of a rapid test, but because the ELISA tests are carried out in batches, rapid tests are cost-effective when small numbers of tests are performed.

Confirming HIV. WHO has recommended strategies for confirming a positive HIV antibody test using combinations of ELISA and simple tests (appendix B, page 199). These strategies mean that it is not necessary to send blood specimens away for the expensive "Western blot" confirmatory test. The strategy varies according to the purpose of the test and the prevalence of infection in the population.

Because these tests are now very sensitive, false positives are a possibility so the strategy for confirming test results is complicated.

Tests for the virus. There are several tests that detect the presence of the virus itself, which are expensive and require sophisticated laboratory support. These include the polymerase chain reaction test (PCR), virus culture, and the antigen test.

The choice of test

The choice of test will depend on the numbers of samples to be tested each day, the cost, storage characteristics, and the sensitivity and specificity of the test.[8] A test that is very sensitive produces few false negatives. A test that is very specific produces few false positives. HIV tests should have a sensitivity greater than 99 percent and a specificity greater than 98 percent (the specificity of test kits may vary according to the geographical origin of the serum samples). Some simple/rapid tests do not require refrigeration and can be stored at temperatures between 2° C and 30° C. Detailed data about ELISA and simple/rapid tests evaluated by WHO are provided in the report "Operational Characteristics of Commercially Available Assays to Determine Antibodies to HIV-1 and/or HIV-2 in Human Sera." This is available from the Blood Safety Unit of WHO.

Be sure that HIV antibody test kits are stored securely, because they have potential to be abused in the wrong hands.

Antibody tests for HIV are expensive. There are a number of strategies to reduce the costs of testing (see appendix B, page 199). Options for recovering the cost of testing by charging clients are not likely to be feasible in humanitarian settings.

Integrating VCT with existing activities

In most humanitarian settings there will not be enough resources to have a dedicated VCT center staffed full-time. There are advantages to integrating VCT services with existing activities, both within and outside health care facilities. Chapter 7 discusses the range of potential

counselors. A VCT service might be available intermittently at youth centers or general information or advice centers. Members of an outreach team that visit clinics could be trained so that VCT is available at intervals to more remote communities.

Promote and distribute condoms

RATIONALE

Promoting and distributing condoms is an important component of preventing sexual transmission of HIV. When people use condoms correctly and consistently they are extremely effective at preventing the spread of STIs, including HIV.

Even if both partners are already infected with HIV there are benefits to using condoms. They prevent exposure to semen and therefore to different strains of the virus and to other STIs; all of these may stimulate white cells to increase viral replication.

Attitudes toward condoms

The group responsible for the condom program needs to be aware of the situation analysis findings in relation to condoms. In order to be able to address people's fears and concerns it is important to understand their attitudes toward condoms.

Many young people have been willing to adopt the use of condoms to protect themselves against infections and pregnancy, and many couples around the world have successfully used condoms to space their families.

But in many settings condoms are still unfamiliar, and many men are reluctant to use them. They may believe that condoms are uncomfortable or reduce pleasure. Young people are often too embarrassed or shy to ask for condoms. Some may not be able to afford condoms, or are unable to obtain them. People often associate condoms with infidelity and immoral behavior. Some do not believe that condoms prevent pregnancy and infections. Some women fear that a condom may get lost inside them. Men and women often find it difficult to talk about sex together. Condoms are used more often during sex outside marriage than inside marriage, and with casual sex more

---

8. "The Importance of Simple/Rapid Assays in HIV Testing Weekly," *Epidemiological Record* 73 (1998): 321–26.

🎗 DISCUSSION POINT 🎗

Role-plays of counseling on radio or TV can be very helpful. It helps people to understand exactly what will happen when they go for VCT. It is also important to have more than one role-play to show a variety of experiences. It is important, however, to make clear that it is a role-play and, to emphasize the importance of confidentiality. In Botswana the Minister of Health was challenged on TV to have an HIV test, and she received her result on TV. This had a powerful effect, with VCT centers reporting large increases in attendance. However, it undermined the minister's right to confidentiality. The lessons are that role-plays of the VCT process are helpful and that personal experiences of well-known people or role models may stimulate people to accept VCT.

What do you think about this? If you cannot prepare a radio role-play perhaps you could prepare a drama or puppet role-play of a VCT session.

---

often than with sex within a long-term or loving relationship. For many people, asking their partner to use a condom suggests a lack of trust. Wives may know that their husbands have sex outside marriage but cannot suggest condoms for fear of abuse or rejection. Another barrier to use is the desire to achieve a pregnancy.

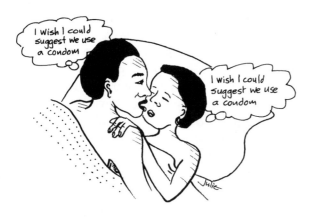

The male condom

The male condom is a thin latex rubber tube that covers the penis during intercourse. Sometimes a condom slips or breaks. Breakage is more common when the condom is too small for the size of the penis. Condoms that are too tight or too short are uncomfortable and might put men off from using condoms.[9] Condoms that are too big may slip off. It is therefore important to order a range of sizes of condoms. There is no evidence that uncircumcised men have more difficulty using condoms than circumcised men. If a condom is stored in a hot place or is past its expiration date it may tear during use. Long fingernails may damage the thin rubber. Oil-based lubricants, such as Vaseline, body lotions, or cooking oil, will damage the latex of the condom within five minutes. It is important to use water-based lubricants such as glycerin, egg white, commercial condom lubricants (e.g., K-Y Jelly), or saliva. In some countries fancy condoms with beads or feathers attached are popular. It is important to communicate the message that these condoms will not protect against infection.

The female condom

The female condom (manufactured by the Female Health Company with trade names: "Reality," "Femidom," and "Care") is like a plastic bag with a flexible ring at each end. A woman inserts the condom before sexual intercourse by squeezing one ring and placing it in

---

9. A. Smith et al., "Factors Affecting Men's Liking of Condoms They Have Used," *International Journal of STD and AIDS* 10 (1999): 258–62.

UNPOPULAR CONDOMS

In Eastern Zaire in 1996 the IRC procured condoms for refugees. It was noted that when clinics were looted during the conflict everything was taken: medicines, needles and syringes, equipment, even the windows. But the boxes of condoms remained untouched. This emphasizes that ordering the condoms is only one component of an effective condom program and highlights the importance of publicity and distribution efforts.

---

position over the cervix. The other ring rests against the vulva outside the vagina.

The female condom is now widely available in many developing countries and is often popular. Unfortunately it is sometimes associated with sex work, but may be a useful option for married women and couples. It is possible to reuse the female condom, although this is not currently recommended by the manufacturer. A laboratory study of the effects of washing, drying, and relubricating female condoms ten times found no significant deterioration in their structural integrity — but it is essential that they be carefully washed and dried to remove any infectious organisms. Advantages include:

- it can be put in place some hours before intercourse, so the woman has some control over her own protection;

- the thin plastic transmits heat so that sex feels more natural than with a male condom;

- oil-based lubricants can be used; and

- sex workers like them because they can continue to work during menstruation.

The disadvantages are:

- it can be difficult to manipulate and insert, especially for inexperienced users;

- it is often noisy during sex;

- the man is able to see and feel the condom;

- it is more expensive than the male condom.

Microbicides

A microbicide is a cream, foam, or gel that is suitable for use in the vagina that will kill HIV and can also reduce the risk of STIs. If these substances cause vaginal inflammation they could increase risk. At present there is no effective microbicide available. Studies of the spermicide nonoxynol-9 suggest that it will not be a useful microbicide. There are a number of substances under investigation at present including a polymer-based "liquid condom" that forms a gel at body temperature. But there are many problems in setting up ethical clinical trials of the efficacy of potential microbicides.

STRATEGIES

Procure adequate numbers of good quality condoms

Condom distribution is an important component of the Minimum Initial Service Package for reproductive health in emergency settings.[10] This is especially important where displaced people have been used to using condoms. However, procurement of condoms does not always mean that they will be distributed and used correctly.

It is possible to contact UNAIDS, UNHCR, UNFPA, or WHO to assist with the purchase of bulk quantities of condoms at low cost.[11] If possible, procure a range of sizes. If men try

10. Inter-Agency Working Group, *Reproductive Health in Refugee Situations: An Inter-Agency Field Manual* (Geneva: UNHCR, 1999).

11. Contact addresses for condom supplies include: IPPF: Regent's College, Inner Circle, Regent's Park, GB-London NW1 4NS, Fax: 44-20-7487; UNFPA: 220 East 42nd Street, New York,

condoms that are too small they may be put off permanently.

Condoms usually come in boxes of 144, called a gross. Quantities may need to be adjusted depending on the situation. You might find that the proportion of the beneficiary population who are sexually active males differs from the assumptions in the formula in the box on page 95. The rate of use of condoms may also vary. To avoid shortages, make sure a three-month reserve supply is available.

There are many brands of condoms on the market. Find out what types of condoms are already available, their quality, and their cost. Is there already any social marketing of condoms in the area? (Social marketing is a process that applies marketing tactics to sell a product or promote a practice with the aim of improving health and well-being). Take care not to undermine existing programs.

Increase accessibility

Consider how to distribute condoms so that they will be accessible to everyone, including the host population. This can best be achieved when condoms are distributed through a variety of channels. Consider all the different groups that may need condoms and how best to reach them. It is especially important to consider how to encourage sexually active young people to use condoms. Free condoms and instructions for use should be available in health care facilities and food distribution centers. They might also be distributed free of charge in workplaces and youth centers. They might be available at low cost through a social marketing program, and sold commercially in hotels, bars, pharmacies, and shops. Consider locating condom outlets where people with high-risk behavior gather. This might be, for example, in military barracks, army shops and canteens, school dormitories, transport centers, truck stops, injecting drug treatment clinics, bars, and commercial sex districts or informal brothels. Peer educators (such as youth, women, sex workers) may also be recruited to

distribute condoms in their communities. If feasible in your setting, condom vending machines provide anonymity as well as convenience and so can improve access.

Social marketing programs have greatly increased access to condoms in many countries. Condoms are heavily promoted through a targeted mass media advertising campaign and sold at a low price, subsidized by donor agencies, such as Population Services International. People sometimes think that free condoms are of lower quality. A high price will put condoms beyond the reach of most people, but a modest cost makes them more valued and likely to be used than if they are free.

Promote condoms

Promoting condoms needs to include efforts to change community attitudes toward condom use and sexual risk-taking. Promotion needs to do more than warn about the risks of AIDS and STIs. It should seek to engage people's interest and persuade them that using condoms is easy, worthwhile, and socially approved.

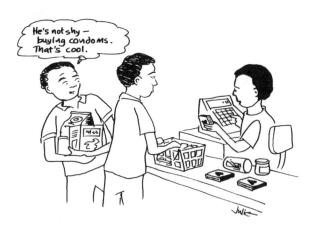

Communication materials can promote an association between condom use and demonstrating care and responsibility, providing peace of mind, and pleasure. Condoms may be promoted for disease prevention or family planning or both, depending on the audience. Women may feel more comfortable talking with their husbands about using condoms for family planning, though they may be more concerned themselves about protection from AIDS. For advice about preparing a community education campaign see page 100.

NY 10017, USA, Fax: 212-297-4915; WHO: Chief, Supplies, CH-1211 Geneva 27, Fax: 41-22-791-41-96.

FORMULA FOR CALCULATING CONDOM REQUIREMENTS

Condom needs can be calculated if you can estimate the following:

- The size of the target population (i.e., refugee/IDP population and adjoining areas). Roughly 20 percent of this number represents the size of the sexually active male population.

- The percentage of males using condoms. Results from previous knowledge, attitudes, behavior, and practices (KAPB) studies can be used when they exist. If they do not exist, plan from data provided by the most reliable source and adapt according to needs.

- Plan for about twelve condoms per sexually active male per month.

- Add 20 percent to the above figure for wastage and loss.

Example:

One month's supply of condoms for an estimated refugee/IDP and adjoining population of 10,000 people, with 20 percent of sexually active males using condoms:

2,000 sexually active males	
20 percent use condoms:	2,000 x 0.2 = 400
12 condoms per month per sexually active male:	400 x 12 = 4,800
Add 20 percent to allow for wastage or loss:	4,800 x 0.2 = 960
Estimated total condom requirements for one month:	**5,760**

—Reproductive Health in Refugee Situations: Inter-Agency Field Manual (1999). *www.rhrc.org/fieldtools/index.htm.*

Catholicism is the religious denomination that has shown the greatest reluctance to promoting the use of condoms to protect against the spread of HIV. However, in April 2000 the Rev. Jacques Suaudeau, of the Pontifical Council for the Family, published an article in the Vatican's official newspaper, *L'Osservatore Romano* (April 19, 2000), indicating that condoms might be permissible for containing the spread of the AIDS virus. The article does not endorse condoms but tolerates their use as part of a comprehensive AIDS education program where the primary emphasis is on moral behavior. He wrote that condoms may be a "lesser evil" than the spread of HIV: "Until a real effort is made [to change their sexual behavior], the prophylactic is one of the best ways to contain the sexual transmission of HIV and AIDS."

Teaching condom skills

Many men feel embarrassed to try using condoms because they do not know what to do. They need to feel confident about their ability to use condoms before they need them. Make sure that instructions are available where condoms are distributed and that staff are trained in how to educate about their use. Counseling and sex education can inform young people and help them to be able to raise the subject of condoms with their partners. Women and girls, as well as men, need to be taught how to put condoms on the penis; this is usually best done one-to-one in a counseling session or in single-sex group education sessions.

The pictures on page 97 can be used in information materials for education sessions on condom use. When teaching people about condoms it can help to have condoms available. They can open the condom to feel how thin the rubber is. They can put a condom over their fingers and feel the eyebrow through the rubber. They can blow up the condom like a balloon to see how strong the rubber is. During post-test counseling or prevention counseling for STI patients, the counselor can rehearse each step of condom use with the client, from buying the condom to disposing of it.

INSTRUCTIONS FOR USE OF CONDOMS

- Do not try to put on the condom when the penis is soft. Put the condom on when the penis has become erect and hard, before the penis touches the partner's genital or anal area.

- Take the condom out of the packet.

- Roll the condom onto the penis.

- Never unroll the condom before use to test it.

- Withdraw the penis soon after ejaculation.

- Hold the condom onto the penis during withdrawal, so that no semen is spilled.

- Tie a knot in the condom and throw it in a latrine or bury it.

- Use a new condom for each act of intercourse.

Strengthen management and control of sexually transmitted infections

RATIONALE

Control of STIs is one of the most effective interventions to reduce HIV transmission.[12]

Some common STIs are gonorrhea, chlamydia, trichomonas, syphilis, chancroid, herpes, and HIV. It is easier for HIV to pass between sexual partners when another STI or other infection of the reproductive tract is present. The risk is much higher when there is an ulcer or sore.

STIs have the same underlying risk factors as HIV. So efforts to prevent the spread of STIs help to prevent the spread of HIV, and the treatment of STI patients presents an opportunity to reach a group at high risk of HIV.

The incidence of STIs varies greatly in different parts of the world, depending on patterns of sexual behavior, susceptibility to infection, and access to health care services. There have been few published studies of STIs among displaced and conflict-affected populations. Studies from Mozambique and Tanzania have shown a high prevalence of STIs and bacterial vaginosis among refugees. The diagnosis and treatment of STIs is inadequate in many parts

of the world and has rarely been given much attention in humanitarian settings.

Women often have no symptoms when infected with gonorrhea or chlamydia, which generally cause a discharge in men. If their sexual partner does not inform them that they may have an infection they will remain unaware. The infection may spread from the vagina or cervix up through the uterus (womb) to the fallopian tubes, and the ovaries to cause acute or chronic pelvic inflammatory disease. The result may be blocked tubes causing infertility or tubal pregnancy. In sub-Saharan Africa 50 percent of cases of infertility are the result of STIs. STIs may also result in cervical cancer and cause miscarriages, stillbirths, low birth weight, prematurity, congenital syphilis, and gonococcal eye infection in the newborn.

The genital sore caused by syphilis will heal by itself if left untreated. Individuals may think that they are clear of the infection. But in fact the syphilis organisms continue to multiply and later cause signs and symptoms throughout the body. This is called secondary syphilis.

Many individuals with symptoms of STIs seek care outside formal health services. This may be because of shame, fear of discrimination, lack of availability of formal health services, cultural beliefs, unwelcoming attitudes of staff, or inability to pay for the treatment. In many countries in Asia and sub-Saharan

---

12. WHO and UNAIDS now tend to use the term "sexually transmitted infections (STIs)" rather than "sexually transmitted diseases (STDs)" because someone may have an STI without having symptoms or signs.

HOW TO USE A CONDOM

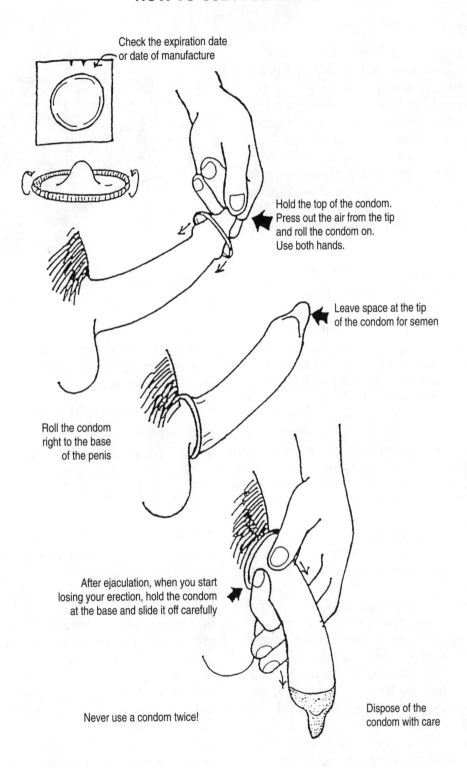

Check the expiration date or date of manufacture

Hold the top of the condom. Press out the air from the tip and roll the condom on. Use both hands.

Leave space at the tip of the condom for semen

Roll the condom right to the base of the penis

After ejaculation, when you start losing your erection, hold the condom at the base and slide it off carefully

Never use a condom twice!

Dispose of the condom with care

Africa, it is common to buy antibiotics from pharmacies. People with STIs may then take an inappropriate antibiotic, or take too short a course, resulting in resistant organisms.

STRATEGIES

To prevent the spread of STIs we need to consider both primary and secondary prevention. Primary prevention aims to change sexual behavior. It includes the encouragement of safer sexual choices, such as abstinence, monogamy, nonpenetrative sex, and consistent use of condoms, and the provision of condoms (see above). Secondary prevention aims to improve access to effective treatment for STIs, to encourage care-seeking behavior, and to detect and treat asymptomatic and symptomatic infections early.

Improving access to effective treatment

A wide variety of services and individuals, both medically qualified and otherwise, provide care for people with STIs. These include STI clinics, hospital outpatient clinics, maternal and child health centers, family planning clinics, private medical practitioners, pharmacies, traditional healers, and street vendors. These can all be sources of information about trends in the rates of STIs and attitudes toward them. Workers in all these settings need training in appropriate management of STIs. The influence of traditional healers can be used to reinforce advice about condom use and reducing the number of sexual partners.

Acceptable and effective STI care needs to be available in a range of settings if it is to be accessible to different groups in the population who have different needs and preferences. For example, STI care integrated with maternal and child health and family planning services is important for enabling women to have asymptomatic STIs detected and to seek treatment for symptoms without fear of stigmatization. But men may not feel comfortable in such women-focused settings, so care for STIs should also be available at primary health care and hospital out-patient clinics. Youth may benefit from health care sessions offered in the evenings in an informal youth center setting and may sometimes prefer to be able to see a doctor or nurse

with one or more friends. Sex workers may be reached through outreach clinics.

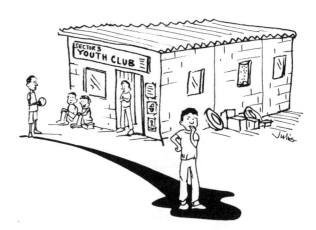

Privacy and confidentiality are essential features for all population groups. The attitudes of staff may prevent people from seeking treatment.

When persons come to a clinic with an STI it is important that they receive comprehensive care. This means that:

- a correct diagnosis is made,
- effective treatment is provided,
- the patient is advised how to take the treatment and for how long,
- future risk-taking behavior by the patient is reduced or prevented,
- condoms are promoted and provided,
- sexual partners are told that they may have an STI and are appropriately treated.

Correct diagnosis

In some settings laboratory services may be available that allow blood tests for syphilis and culture of swabs for gonorrhea and chlamydia. New DNA tests enable diagnosis of STIs from urine or tampon specimens. Where such services are not available there may be a microscope that allows for simple observation for gonorrhea (using a gram stain) or trichomonas. Simple serological testing for syphilis is recommended for case finding in pregnant women and screening of blood donors.

Often, however, health care workers need to rely on syndromic management, where the choice of treatment depends on the particular pattern of signs and symptoms. For example, for the syndrome "vaginal discharge" they treat for gonorrhea, trichomonas, and chlamydia. Syndromic diagnosis avoids wrong diagnoses and ineffective treatment, can be learned by primary health workers, and allows treatment of symptomatic patients in one visit. However, it cannot assist in the management of asymptomatic infections and means that patients may take medicines for STIs that they do not have.

The flow charts for syndromic management of STIs appear in appendix D (page 207).

Effective treatment

The specific choice of treatment will depend on local antibiotic sensitivity studies and availability of antibiotics. Whenever possible the choice of antibiotics should be consistent with national treatment protocols. For effective treatment to be possible health care workers need to be well trained in syndromic management, and antibiotics need to be appropriately ordered and stored. Patients need specific advice about how to take the treatment and for how long. As services and awareness improve, expect a rapid increase in the amounts of antibiotics required.

In Uganda pre-packaged treatment kits have been introduced for male urethral discharge.[13] The kits contain the antibiotics ciprofloxacin and doxycycline, condoms, partner referral cards, and patient information. They have been socially marketed with success. The kits are popular with patients but not with health workers who may feel that they lose their role when people can buy treatment without a consultation. But in places where well-informed counseling is not available and people are literate these kits may well be a valuable strategy in the management and control of STIs.

Prevention counseling

When patients attend with an STI this is an opportunity to counsel them about the risk of HIV infection. If HIV testing is available this should be offered to them. Condoms need to be available in all clinics to offer to patients with STIs.

Contact tracing (partner notification)

Contact tracing means finding and telling the partner/s of a person with an STI that they might be infected and should be treated. The aim is to:

- treat all sexual partners (within the past three months, at least) of the STI patient;
- treat the partners for the same STI.

This should be done in a way that maintains confidentiality and is not compulsory. Counseling and support should be available.

Contact tracing is always difficult, but it is likely to be even more difficult to carry out in a humanitarian setting. Although in a camp setting it may be easier to contact partners, it is unlikely that many patients will be willing to identify their sexual partners. However, contact tracing is a very effective way to reduce the spread of STIs in a community so it is worth considering whether it would be feasible to introduce any of the systems described below.

Because women often have no symptoms when they have an STI, it is particularly important to try to contact and treat the female partners of male STI patients.

There are several ways to contact partners:

1. **Patient referral:** The health care worker asks patients to tell their partners to come for examination and treatment. They do not ask for information about the partners. Patients may receive contact cards or referral slips to give to their sexual partner/s.

   In some places the health care workers give the patient medicines to give to their partners. If health care workers refuse to treat patients unless they bring their partners, this might discourage people with STIs from attending the clinic for treatment.

2. **Health care worker referral:** The health care worker obtains names and contact details of sexual partners and tries

---

13. For more information contact The Futures Group International, *www.tfgi.com/.*

to contact them by visiting, mail, or telephone.

3. **Patient and health care worker referral:** The health care worker asks for names and contact details of partners, but gives patients time to ask them themselves. If they do not appear for treatment, health care workers try to contact them.

Encouraging care-seeking behavior

The above measures to improve access to effective STI treatment will encourage care-seeking behavior. A community education campaign, targeted to those most vulnerable to STIs, such as young people, the military, and clients of sex workers, can also encourage attendance. Such a campaign will be more effective if those targeted are involved in designing the materials, and if the messages and media are based on an understanding of the barriers to seeking care.

Detecting and treating asymptomatic and symptomatic infections early

Detecting asymptomatic infections is not possible without laboratory diagnostic services. Where these are not available health workers need to be trained in syndromic management and in treating women who have reason to fear that they have been exposed to an STI, even though they do not have symptoms. Community education and the chance to be seen in private by a female health worker who is nonjudgmental will encourage women to attend for screening and treatment. The management of women who have been raped or sexually assaulted should include screening for STIs. Testing for syphilis, and treatment if required, should be a routine part of prenatal care whenever possible. If the prevalence of syphilis is known to be 10 percent or greater, consider treating all pregnant women with a single injection of benzathine penicillin at the first prenatal visit.

An STI increases the risk of HIV transmission from an HIV-infected mother to her child, so it is especially important to screen for and treat STIs promptly during pregnancy and to promote condom use. Sex workers also need access to nonjudgmental health care services;

an outreach service by a trusted health worker can increase the likelihood of early diagnosis and treatment.

Surveillance

The situation analysis should reveal whether there are local, provincial, or national STI surveillance systems in place. A service for refugees and IDPs should become part of such a system if feasible. If possible try to obtain a baseline assessment of the prevalence of STIs through a population-based survey.

INTERVENTIONS THAT RELATE TO CHANGING INDIVIDUAL BEHAVIORS

Develop and disseminate communication materials for behavior change[14]

Information, Education, and Communication (IEC) is a jargon term, but it can be a useful way to describe a necessary component of the overall response to HIV. We know that information alone is insufficient to achieve behavior change or reduce people's vulnerability. Nevertheless information is necessary, and communication campaigns can certainly raise awareness and change attitudes. Commercial companies allocate a large part of their budget to advertising because they know that it is effective in persuading people to buy a particular product or service. A lot of this budget is spent on market research in order to understand the characteristics of the audience that they want to target and their attitudes, beliefs, and practices in relation to the product or service. Their market research helps them to make decisions about the messages, the media, and the types of appeal that they will use to reach particular groups. Advertisements are always pre-tested and modified before being displayed or broadcast.

AIDS prevention activities in the past have often focused narrowly on the production of information materials such as posters and pamphlets. In order to emphasize the aim of achieving behavior change and the need for

---

14. Much of this section is adapted from A. Starrs and R. Rizzuto, *Getting the Message Out: Designing an Information Campaign on Women's Health* (New York: Family Care International, 1995).

broader communication strategies the term "behavior change communication" (BCC) was introduced. Many activities described in the various chapters of this manual are part of "behavior change communication."

It is challenging to carry out a communication campaign in a refugee/IDP setting. But in the post-emergency phase it may be possible, and there may be additional benefits such as providing purposeful activity and much needed entertainment through the development of appropriate folk media. It may be possible to make use of materials already in use in the refugees' country of origin. But bear in mind that sensitivities may have changed with the population's changed circumstances, so that old messages may no longer be appropriate or effective. It will be difficult to engage people who are fatalistic with little optimism for the future.

Many interventions need the support of a communication campaign. For example IEC is an important part of a condom promotion and distribution intervention. It can make people aware of the availability and benefits of a new service such as VCT and help to alter discriminatory attitudes before prenatal VCT testing is introduced. IEC materials can assist peer educators in their work.

Communication programs are most useful when they are interactive or stimulate responses from the community. It is important when planning communication campaigns to think about their timing in relation to other initiatives, especially activities that allow opportunities for community discussions. Look for opportunities to convey messages related to HIV prevention and care through existing activities. Perhaps a relevant video might be shown in a youth center, a singing group could perform songs that reinforce caring and nonjudgmental attitudes, or a literacy group could prepare posters with simple messages.

All three components of IEC need to be taken into account in planning:

- information (accurate facts about the topic),

- education (understanding and making meaning of the information in a given context),

- communication (interaction between people to enable understanding to occur).

Information must be accurate, clear, and at an appropriate language level. To increase understanding people need opportunities to talk with others about the information. One of the most powerful communication strategies is "word of mouth" or "friend to friend" conversations. The speed at which rumors spread is evidence of this. Unfortunately misinformation can also spread in this way. Understanding and using informal communication networks is valuable in promoting dialogue.

In planning a communication campaign you first need to think about the interests and needs of the different kinds of people you want to reach — that is, the target groups. "Target groups" might be those at higher risk, such as young people, sex workers, military personnel, drivers, or those who inject drugs. But take care not to stigmatize or offend these groups, for example, by obviously targeting them in posters viewed by all. Communication campaigns are more likely to be effective if the target groups themselves help to design and deliver them. Target groups may also be segments of the population divided by sex, age, occupations, or beliefs. It is generally more cost-effective to appeal separately to different groups than to try to reach everyone in the same way.

You then need to think about the special information that each group needs and how to present it to them in a meaningful way. So you have to think about the messages and the media, or channels, that will be used to communicate the message.

Whatever the specific objective of the communication campaign, the working group, which should include members of the targeted groups, will need to review the relevant findings from the situation analysis.

Content of messages

The content of the messages needs to include:

- information that the different target groups need to have but don't have now,

- actions that the target groups need to take but are not yet taking,

- suggestions for overcoming obstacles that may stop them from taking an action that they have decided they want to take.

Media or channels of communication

In order to choose appropriate channels of communication you need to know how to reach the target groups. The situation analysis report should provide information about the ways that the target groups get information. You also need to think about which media and which method of distribution might be appropriate for the specific messages. It is always best to use a variety of media.

There are six main types of communication channels:

1. Mass media. Mass media campaigns (newspapers, magazines, radio, and television) are able to reach large numbers. Mass media can help to raise awareness but alone may not influence people to change their behavior. Mass campaigns can have a harmful effect if they are conducted before supportive services are available. For example, it is no use promoting condoms if they are not available or alarming people about AIDS if there are no counselors. A mass campaign may result in misinformation if there are no sources of further information and explanation. Health workers need to be aware of programs on the radio and articles in newspapers about AIDS so that they know what their patients may have heard or read.

In the settings in which NGOs work radio may be the most widely available and popular form of mass communication. Radio programs are not expensive to produce, are convincing, and reach people who cannot read. When the programs are entertaining, relevant to people's lives, and informative, they often stimulate discussion with friends and relatives. Radio can be a useful tool in raising awareness for behavior change and in maintaining commitment. It is helpful to include in the situation analysis questions about how many people own radios, who listens, how often, and at what times of day. What programs do people of different ages and gender prefer? What different types of radio channels are there? Do people trust the information they hear on the radio?

Different styles of program appeal to different age groups and genders; they also listen at different times of day. Consider preparing a simple fact sheet on AIDS as background material for radio announcers.

Newsletters and magazines may include articles about health or sex. They sometimes have very useful articles about HIV. They can explain "safer sex" in more detail than is acceptable on TV or radio or in newspapers. But magazines are expensive, and like TV they may reach only a small proportion of the population. Young people might like to produce their own "magazine," including articles that promote sexual health, which could be copied and passed around among young people.

Mass media can also be interactive — through letters or telephone if available. A simple quiz competition with a prize in a newspaper or newsletter can be an effective way to engage people and convey information.

2. Print media. Print media include:

- publications for reading, such as pamphlets, leaflets, brochures, and booklets;

- materials for display, such as posters, calendars, and wall charts; and

- materials for use with individuals or groups, such as flip charts and picture cards.

Leaflets and brochures are useful for people who can read. They can contain information which might be embarrassing, and the client can take it away to study privately. Leaflets can give detailed information and remind a client about important points from a counseling session. They can include pictures or diagrams and can be shared and discussed to spread the information and gain the support and understanding of others.

Flip-charts and brochures can help health workers and counselors to give accurate information without forgetting important points.

By themselves, posters have little value because they can provide only brief information. They cannot explain details of safe sex practices, for example. However, they can draw attention to a topic, and they can reinforce a message that the public receives through other media. They can provide a point for discussion.

A "picture code" is a poster-sized illustration that can be used to present a familiar problem about which a community or group has strong feelings, in order to stimulate discussion and suggestions for solutions.[15]

Some tips for designing print media:

- Print media should be in the local language.

- Use large type that will be easy to read. Try to avoid CAPITALS and *italics;* studies show that these are more difficult to read. Use only one font or style.

- Use simple but precise words and short sentences.

- Make sure that colors used are acceptable and do not have inappropriate meanings for the refugee/IDP or local population.

- Try to make any pictures realistic and include familiar objects.

- Always include information about where to get more detailed information and advice.

It is important to think about how people who are not literate or do not understand the local language may interpret materials such as pamphlets and posters. For example, a pamphlet may use illustrations to show both how HIV is and is not transmitted. To someone who cannot read the explanation it may appear as though HIV spreads through mosquitoes and sharing plates and cups.

Similarly it is important to be careful that pictures used to illustrate routes of transmission are clear and not open to misinterpretation. For example, a picture of a couple embracing might suggest that HIV spreads through hugging rather than through sexual intercourse. This adds to stigmatization. Of course it is difficult to illustrate sexual intercourse in a way that is both unambiguous and acceptable. Think about whether there are symbols that might be appropriate to use and easily recognized by the population. For example, in China, the magpie is the Bird of Joy, and two magpies represent "marital bliss" or "happy sex"; in some countries a picture of an empty double bed might

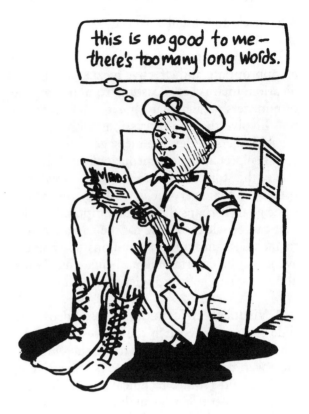

be appropriate. But all such images need pre-testing to check how they will be understood by a variety of audiences.

3. Folk media. Traditional forms of communication and entertainment include theater, storytelling, songs, dance, poems, puppet shows, and messages displayed on cloth or clothing. They have a useful place in refugee/IDP settings because they bring many people together in traditional and familiar ways.

Puppets can introduce sensitive topics, such as death and sex, and they can portray what people think and do without causing offense or embarrassment. Puppets can criticize, use humor, try out solutions, and show difficulties that people face.

A puppet show is most likely to be effective if the target group is involved in both development and performance. Follow it with a small group discussion that enables people to relate what they have heard about AIDS to their own lives. Puppets cost little to make, but to organize a puppet show takes time and enthusiasm. Puppet shows and drama can reach remote areas that mass media cannot. Use local

---

15. S. Laver, *Let's Teach about AIDS,* Healthlink Worldwide.

references and familiar place names in your stories.

In some countries religious sermons might be an appropriate and effective means of communication. Imams broadcasting from the mosque or ministers preaching in church can be influential. Involve them in discussions with community members to develop messages.

When preparing folk media make a clear outline of the story and messages that you want to present so that everyone is working toward the same goal. Perhaps there are traditional stories that can provide the base for the narrative. Try to include a mixture of emotions so that the event will be entertaining and engaging. Think about ways to get the audience to join in.

4. Visual electric media. Films, videos, and slide shows easily catch the interest of people who rarely have the chance to see such images. However, these media can be very expensive to produce and require technical skills. Unless a portable generator is available they cannot be used where there is no electricity. It is best to use these media as a discussion starter, with a trained facilitator who has a discussion guide. There are several videos that tell a story or present case studies or documentaries related to AIDS. Try to find out whether there are any in appropriate languages.

Images or slides of clinical manifestations of AIDS may be very useful to train health care workers on how to recognize clinical signs in their patients. But be careful when using these slides, especially if they are graphic. Such pictures should not be used to "scare" people into safer sex. They can be upsetting, may increase stigma, and can result in young people associating sex with disease.

5. Special events. Special events might include competitions, games, parades, rallies, and launches of new projects or activities. Social events or awareness-raising days can provide an opportunity to use a range of media to get messages out. Make sure that you consult carefully before choosing the date. Allow plenty of time for consultation and planning. Allocate resources and time for publicity so that you get maximum coverage for your event. Ask

local celebrities to become involved. Don't forget to arrange some activities that children can participate in.

6. Personal or community counseling. Direct contact with a health worker or counselor can make people decide to change their behavior. It can give them a sense of personal risk. This contact may be individual, during consultations for other purposes, or in groups at a community level. Health workers need to be trained in communication skills. They need to become confident at starting to talk with the community, at showing respect, and in listening skills. Refer to chapter 7 on counseling, and to guides on communication skills.[16]

Try to identify people in the community who have a lot of contact with people, such as hairdressers or barbers, who could be trained to provide information about AIDS. They have an opportunity to talk with people privately and may also be in a position to distribute or sell condoms. In Vietnam cyclo drivers were trained as peer educators because they often take men to sex workers. But the drivers often found it difficult to initiate a conversation about AIDS and condoms despite having good knowledge. Provide suggestions and role-play practice for ways to start a conversation about AIDS.

Choosing the appeal

The appeal is the approach that the material uses to attract attention and influence people, such as fear, humor, or emotion.

Because of the fatal nature of AIDS, it is tempting to try to frighten people into changing their behavior. The skeleton is probably one of the most common images used in AIDS information campaigns! Health educators can learn from studies by market researchers. These studies show that messages that are too frightening produce psychological barriers. Fear may cause people to notice only part of the message or make people believe that the message does not apply to them. People may laugh off or deny a frightening message. Fear of AIDS together

---

16. Jill Tabbutt, *Strengthening Communication Skills for Women's Health: A Training Guide* (New York: Family Care International, 1995).

DISCUSSION POINT

What do you think about mixing religious or moral messages with health messages?

When you facilitate this discussion make sure that several religions are discussed rather than focusing on a single religion. Encourage people to speak with respect for other's beliefs.

Some points to consider:

Changes in hygiene behavior are important to prevent the spread of many infectious diseases. Hygiene practices certainly have sensitive cultural aspects, and there are strong attitudes and beliefs connected with them. Nevertheless, religions do not generally mix moral messages with health messages in relation to the prevention of diarrhea and trachoma. It is safer to wash your hands before you eat and to wash your children's faces—but you are not considered a sinner if you do not do these things. But in relation to sexual behavior it is common for the messages to be mixed. Religious leaders sometimes use health messages to reinforce their teaching of morals. They may say to young people: "If you remain abstinent and do not sin then you will not contract HIV or STIs." "If you are unfaithful to your wife you are sinning and you may get HIV." One unfortunate effect of this is that when someone has HIV others will think that they have sinned. The messages stigmatize the disease.

Sometimes people with strong religious beliefs will not promote certain methods to protect against spread of the virus, even though they may be effective, because they believe that they are morally wrong. For example, Catholics may be unwilling to teach that using condoms will reduce the risk of HIV transmission during sex. They may also be unwilling to teach young people that masturbation and nonpenetrative sexual activity are safe ways to enjoy their sexuality and express love without risking pregnancy, STIs, and HIV infection.

On the other hand religious leaders might argue that it is very difficult to change behavior—and that love or fear of God may be a strong motivating factor that helps people to change. Appeals to people's sense of responsibility to care for each other may challenge stigma and increase care and support for people with AIDS.

Church groups or religious organizations are often important structures within the community. They often provide support and welfare services and are well placed to coordinate home-based care and orphan support services.

with ignorance can encourage misunderstandings about who is at risk and why. Fear may be one cause of the stigma attached to AIDS patients.

Humor can reduce the tension that may arise when people discuss serious and sensitive topics.

Educated people may respond to messages based on facts and figures, but you do not have to give details about the virus or the immune system to justify safer sex advice. Refer to ideas of disease and family values that people in the community already understand.

Pre-testing materials and ideas

Understandings of disease and human behavior vary greatly. It is easy for messages to be misunderstood. HIV/AIDS is a particularly difficult disease for people to understand. Try out drafts of leaflets or other material with people from the target group to find out if they can understand and respond.

- Do they agree with the information?
- Do they find it easy to understand?
- Do they find it offensive?
- Do they think the advice applies to them?

You can use in-depth interviews and focus group discussions for pre-testing materials (see page 44). Try to talk with different people from those who were interviewed during the situation analysis. It is especially important to avoid leading questions because you want to know what people have understood from the materials. Often several rounds of pre-testing are necessary. Test early drafts, make modifications, and test again.

Production and distribution

Once the messages and media have been pre-tested and finalized they need to be distributed. Communication materials cannot be effective sitting on a shelf.

If you have materials that need to be printed, find out whether others in your setting have had things printed and find out where they did so. If you are in a position to choose, obtain quotes from different printers. Make sure that copyright issues are clear. You might need to

discuss this in the team if several organizations are involved. Who has ownership of the materials? Remember always to get permission when you take and use photographs. If you are showing people with HIV they should either not be recognizable or they should be identified by name with their permission. If you use pictures from other publications, check whether you need to get permission from the publisher. Many books produced for developing countries give permission for pictures and text to be copied or adapted, but they appreciate receiving copies of such materials.

Think carefully and consult about the best places to put posters and brochures. Consider distribution points, markets, churches, sports venues, youth centers, and clinics. Try to make sure that posters are protected from wind and rain. Ask permission to place them inside buildings.

Train health workers or volunteers in the use of flip charts and brochures.

Post-production

It is important to monitor and evaluate responses to the communication campaign, make appropriate revisions, and seek new ideas.

Some hazards in choosing HIV/AIDS education messages: Information about AIDS without discussion can increase stigma, especially when the messages are designed to frighten people and the routes of transmission are presented in a way that associates them in people's minds with bad or immoral behavior.

Be wary of using terms that may have different meanings to different people. For example don't label people as "heterosexual" or "homosexual," or as "sex workers," but find out about people's own definitions and identities.

Don't forget that older people have sex too, and in refugee/IDP settings they may have lost their partners and seek new partners. Include some older people, both men and women, in pictures or songs.

The term "innocent victims" is often used when referring to children with HIV. Avoid this term because it implies that other people with HIV are "guilty." The word "victims" makes people with HIV sound passive. It is better to use the expression: "People living with HIV."

Messages such as "You get AIDS from having multiple partners" or "Don't be promiscuous" mislead as well as result in stigma. In many countries the majority of women infected with HIV have only had one sexual partner — their husband. Women are unlikely to be willing to learn about HIV or admit to knowing about HIV when it has been so closely associated with socially unacceptable sexual behavior. Women who may be infected will be reluctant to be tested or to disclose their infection because they will be thought by others to be promiscuous. The message contributes to stigma and discrimination and adds to the risk that people infected with HIV will be rejected by their families.

HIV/AIDS has several features that make it a difficult disease for people to understand. You might want to review the discussion about this on page 72 when preparing information materials.

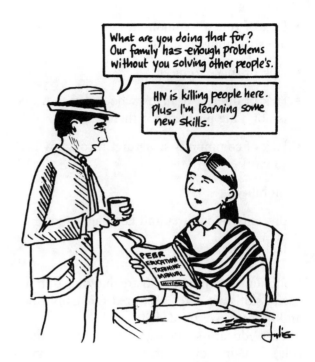

Promote peer education

Peer educators can be effective at disseminating information and influencing behavior. It is a cost-effective strategy that is likely to be feasible in humanitarian settings and can be readily incorporated into existing activities. Groups from whom peers may be recruited and trained include married women, youth, and workplace colleagues. The peer education strategy can be especially useful with groups that may be difficult to reach such as sex workers, men who have sex with men, and injecting drug users.

Advantages

Peer educators may be able to incorporate their HIV awareness messages into their daily work and activities. They may have several roles — disseminating information, distributing condoms, or supervising "directly observed short course therapy" for tuberculosis patients (DOTS). They may also play the role of facilitators in community group discussions. Peer educators may be given resources to develop their own ideas. They may be able to reach large numbers of people through extensive informal networks.

Being a peer educator can increase confidence and self-esteem, encourage a sense of ownership of the program, and provide useful skills to community volunteers. Peer educators can also play a useful role in advocacy work, since they become aware through their work of the needs of their peers.

Support

Although a peer education strategy is relatively inexpensive, it does need to be adequately resourced if it is to be effective. A system for coordination, supervision, and support needs to be established. Peer educators need to be well trained in one-to-one health education and counseling so that they feel equipped to provide support if needed. They need to be able to refer people with problems or illness. For example, if women peer educators raise the awareness of other women about the need to get treatment for STIs, they need to have somewhere to refer them when they do complain of symptoms. It is important not to exploit volunteer peer educators or treat them as though they were paid workers. Peer educators can keep logbooks to keep a record of their contacts with community members.

Constraints

Peer educators often face difficulties that lead to frustration and high turnover:

- lack of time of community members who are struggling to survive,

- lack of space to meet,

- lack of interest of many who feel that AIDS is not a big problem for them,

- lack of community structures through which to work,

- mobility,

- diversity of cultures and language, and

- lack of literacy.

Community members who are outgoing or have useful skills are often recruited for many roles and become overburdened.

Peer educators often gain status from their role, but in some settings adolescent girls trained as peer educators have been stigmatized by their families and communities. Knowledge about sex and reproduction is often hidden from girls until they marry. Some may believe that these young girls have acquired their knowledge through experience rather than through training, and so they may be rejected. It is important that these peer educators remain associated with and supported by the program team. The subject matter of training should be broad so that public perception is not that peer educators have been trained only in sex. For example, training in child health could usefully be included in the "curriculum" for young peer educators. Youth peer educators might be linked with adult peer educators for support.

Encouragement

Encouragement for peer educators might take the form of T-shirts, practical help, for example, with sewing classes or schoolwork, or small cash allowances. Motivation can be maintained by putting peer educators into contact with other peer educators — perhaps through an electronic mailing list. The opportunity to attend a conference and meet other peer educators can provide great encouragement and enable them to see the significance of their role in a wider context.

Provide sex education for young people

Young people learn about sex and sexuality in every society. They may learn from parents, aunts, and uncles, or through sex education in schools. Some societies leave young people to find out about sexuality through trial and error on their own, from friends, or from films, magazines, books, and advertisements. Where people have been displaced young people may miss out on any information about sex and sexuality. Yet they are likely to be especially vulnerable to the hazards of early sexual activity and sexual exploitation.

Sexual health

It is very important for girls and boys to have knowledge about how their bodies work and change during puberty. If they understand about sex and relationships, they will be in a better position to protect themselves from harm and to enjoy good sexual health throughout their lives. The World Health Organization describes sexual health as "the integration of the physical, emotional, intellectual and social aspects of sexual being, in ways that are enriching and that enhance personality, communication and love."

In some places sex education in schools is more than simply a lesson in biology. Children learn about self-confidence, respect, and relationships as well as the facts about sex. Studies show that sex education for young people does not make them more likely to have sex at an early age. In fact it often helps girls to have the confidence and communication skills to say no to boys who pressure them to have sex against their wishes.[17]

It is best to emphasize the positive benefits of safer behavior and suggest different and safer ways to express sexuality. Attempts to frighten young people into not having sex at all are not effective. They may react to fear by denying that there is a problem. It is natural for young people to enjoy taking risks. Also, linking sex with death and disease can

---

17. "Lessons from 'Auntie Stella': Using PRA to Promote Reproductive Health Education in Zimbabwe's Secondary Schools," *PLA Notes* 37 (February 2000).

have bad effects on young people's future relationships and prevent them from fully enjoying sex. Help them to develop communication and assertion skills, and try to increase their self-esteem. Some youth are full of false confidence and believe that they are immune to disaster. On the other hand young people may believe that all their peers are having sex, so it may be important to emphasize that many young people prefer to choose to wait until they are older before they have sex. Adolescents are often very aware of their bodies. This may show itself by interest in grooming or in sport. Stress their responsibility to protect their bodies.

There is a need to understand local attitudes toward what are thought of as desirable characteristics for sexual intercourse. For example, in some countries well-lubricated sex is generally thought to be more desirable than dry sex. But in many countries girls are taught to use a variety of substances, such as leaves, herbs, and various powders, to dry and tighten their vaginas, because there is a perception that men prefer "dry" sex. It is important to teach girls that it is healthy to wash the external genitals, but that there is no need to wash inside their vagina because it is a self-cleaning organ. They need to know that putting chemicals or herbs in the vagina may cause inflammation that predisposes to infections, including possibly infection with HIV. Boys also need to be taught about the importance of washing their genitals and that it is normal and natural for a woman to have slippery vaginal secretions if she is relaxed and sexually excited.

Sex education in school

Research shows that AIDS education targeted at young people before they become sexually active is most successful in minimizing future risk behavior. The school setting is the most obvious in which to reach young people, but class teachers may not be the most appropriate people to deliver AIDS education in a sensitive way. Some students prefer to discuss sexual behavior with an anonymous person rather than with their teacher. Some classroom teachers may feel uncomfortable, uncertain, and embarrassed when they talk with their students about sexual practices.

Your strategic plan might include training teachers and providing them with resources to assist them to teach children about sex and HIV infection. It is important to be aware that there may be resistance to the idea of sex education in schools from parents and education officials. If you can talk to them first about the risks of HIV infection, it may help you to obtain their approval. Consulting parents about what to teach their children about AIDS may also help.

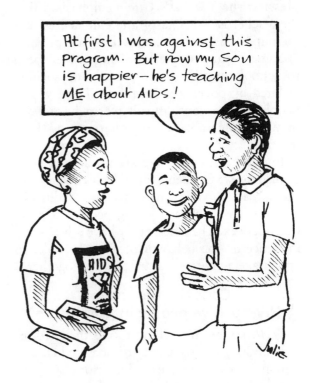

Methods

Learning methods that lead young people to make their own decisions are more effective than lectures. Small group discussions in privacy can lead young people to explore their own feelings and values. Teachers might use games, role-play, puppets, songs, and drama. Talks by people living with HIV are very effective ways to personalize the risk for young people.

The popularity of "problem aunties" in magazines led to an idea for an effective method of sex education for young people in schools in Zimbabwe. "Auntie Stella" consists of cards with questions supposedly written by adolescents seeking advice about a range of sexual health–related topics. There are corresponding cards with Auntie Stella's replies. Young people discuss the "problem" cards in small single-sex groups, guided by "talking points" that follow the problem letter. Then they look at and discuss the "answer cards," which include "action points." This has been found to be very effective because adolescents are most at ease when talking to peers of the same sex, but feel inhibited in full-class discussion and in discussions with the opposite sex, especially if a teacher is present. The *Teacher's Guide* emphasizes that the teacher is a facilitator and emphasizes that the pupils' discussions and writing are private.

Some young people who have never been to school may be geographically or socially isolated by poverty or disability. These young people can be very difficult to reach, and yet may be vulnerable to exploitation and HIV infection.

In many societies there are traditional rules governing sexual behavior, which can prevent the spread of HIV. There may be traditional methods to encourage young people to practice safer sex. The elderly may have a beneficial influence on the behavior of young people, so encourage activities that bring them together.

Consider the role of HIV-positive people in prevention

PLWH/As who are willing to tell their stories publicly are able to change attitudes, reduce discrimination, and encourage behavior change by personalizing vulnerability to infection. Many people believe that it is possible to tell that a person has HIV by their appearance. PLWH/A who look healthy challenge this false belief. When people with HIV/AIDS speak out in public they challenge stereotypes about who becomes infected. It also increases tolerance and understanding toward PLWH/A. When people meet PLWH/A, they feel able to talk more openly about AIDS and the social and sexual issues that increase its spread. But there can be adverse effects for those who speak out; PLWH/A should never be pressured to disclose their infection as a service to the general community (see chapter 10).[18]

----

18. S. Paxton, *Lifting the Burden of Secrecy: A Manual for HIV-Positive People Who Want to Speak Out in Public* (Asia-Pacific Network of People Living with HIV/AIDS, October 1999).

Provide prevention counseling for STI patients

When patients seek treatment for an STI there is an excellent opportunity to counsel them about behavior change and provide condoms (see page 91).

INTERVENTIONS THAT RELATE TO THE SOCIETAL CONTEXT

Efforts to increase the community's capacity to create an enabling environment for behavior change and to reduce vulnerability to HIV presents a challenge in humanitarian settings.

Often the refugees or IDPs gathered in a camp, living among a host community, or living in resettled villages were originally members of several different communities, possibly on opposing sides in the conflict. They may have different values and beliefs. Even where all are from a single community the social fabric is likely to have been torn by displacement, with community leaders missing, the usual composition of the community disturbed, community structures damaged, and social rituals interrupted.

Community development initiatives in these circumstances are not impossible, but there are likely to be frequent setbacks. The need to restore dignity and trust is great.

Where refugees and IDPs have been living together for years, community structures and relationships will have evolved and the setting will have more similarity to a stable community. Nevertheless the nature of life for a displaced person is temporary, and if there are changes in their place of origin that make returning home feasible, they will leave. Community development initiatives often imply a long-term commitment and permanence. For this reason such initiatives may be resented or opposed by both the refugees/IDPs and the host government and population.

Prevent and manage the consequences of sexual and gender-based violence

This is a difficult issue to study, but wherever attempts have been made to document sexual and gender-based violence it has been found to be extremely common during armed conflicts and in displaced populations. In the early phases of a conflict rape is most likely by unknown men and soldiers, while in the post-emergency phase rape and coerced sex are more likely to be by men known to the woman. Domestic violence seems to be common in all settings, and there is evidence that it is also common in humanitarian settings, where men may have high levels of frustration, powerlessness, and boredom. In a camp with Somali and Sudanese refugees in northern Kenya, 12 percent of women surveyed said they had been hit by someone in their home in the past month.

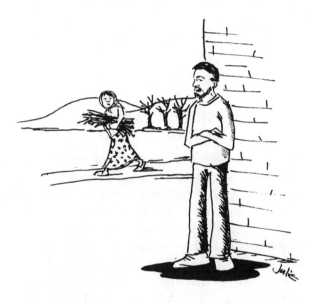

In addition to the risk of HIV, sexual and gender-based violence has other serious consequences. Survivors often experience depression, terror, guilt, shame, and loss of self-esteem. Rejection by families can further increase their vulnerability to exploitation. They may also suffer from unwanted pregnancy, unsafe abortions, STIs, sexual dysfunction, trauma to the reproductive tract, and chronic infections leading to pelvic inflammatory disease and infertility.[19]

Rape and sexual assault violate the victims' rights to privacy and integrity of the person. The UN Commission on Human Rights passed

the first resolution to identify rape as a war crime in 1993. The conviction for rape of three soldiers at the war-crimes tribunal in The Hague in March 2001 was an important step in undermining the culture of impunity. In local settings advocacy for publicizing and applying penalties for rape and domestic violence are also essential in order to raise awareness and shift community attitudes.

Men may also be subjected to rape and sexual assault, especially in captivity. It may be even more difficult for them to disclose this than for women. Children too may be vulnerable to sexual abuse.

But protecting against sexual and gender-based violence is a difficult challenge. There is much greater awareness now among NGOs, and preventing and managing the consequences of sexual violence are key components of the Minimum Initial Service Package for reproductive health in humanitarian settings.

Measures for assisting displaced and conflict-affected persons who have experienced sexual violence, including rape, must be established in the early phase of an emergency. The UNHCR Guidelines for Prevention and Response to Sexual Violence against Refugees (1995) should be followed. Women who have experienced sexual violence should be referred to the health services as soon as possible after the incident. Key actions to be taken during the emergency to reduce the risk of sexual violence and respond to survivors are:

- design and locate refugee/IDP camps, in consultation with refugees/IDPs, to enhance physical security;

- ensure the presence of female protection and health staff and interpreters;

- include women in the distribution of shelter, food, and other supplies;

- include the issues of sexual violence in the health coordination meetings;

- ensure communities are informed of the availability of services for survivors of sexual violence;

- provide a medical response to survivors of sexual violence, including emergency contraception, as appropriate;

19. S. Krause, R. Jones, and S. Purdin, "Programmatic Responses to Refugees' Reproductive Health Needs," *International Family Planning Perspectives* 26 (2000): 181–87.

RAPE AND ECONOMICS

In a population of 106,000 refugees in Dadaab, Kenya, 106 cases of rape were reported in the first nine months of 1998, more than in all of 1997. Researchers discovered that the refugees attributed increased sexual violence to worsening security and to lack of economic opportunity for women. Economic security would allow women to buy firewood rather than collect it in unsafe areas outside the camp, where more than 90 percent of rapes were said to occur, and also would allow them to resist demands for sex from other refugees and authorities within the camp.

— S. Olila, S. Igras, and B. Monahan, "Assessment Report: Issues and Responses to Sexual Violence, Dadaab Refugee Camps, Kenya, 16–23 Oct. 1998," Nairobi, Kenya, and Atlanta, Georgia, USA: CARE.

- identify individuals or groups who may be particularly at risk of sexual violence (single female heads-of-households, unaccompanied minors, etc.) and address their protection and assistance needs.[20]

In the post-emergency setting protection involves both practical measures and assisting the community to develop their own responses and change attitudes. This requires exploration of gender relations. Planning practical measures for protection needs to involve community leaders, men and women, to avoid well-intentioned mistakes. For example, toilets may be well lit to try to prevent attacks, but women may not be able to use them because modesty demands that they use toilets only when they will not be seen.

We recommend that you refer to the *Inter-Agency Manual of Reproductive Health in Refugee Settings,* which has a useful chapter on preventing and managing sexual violence in the post-emergency setting. Here we present only the summary checklist for sexual violence programs.

Provide opportunities for social activities

In addition to protecting women from forced or coerced sex there is a need to create opportunities for men and women to meet in culturally acceptable ways.[21] Social activities should not be viewed as a luxury, secondary to the essentials of shelter, water, and food, but as necessary to restore the community's rights to dignity. Such activities can restore morale, a sense of trust, and hope for the future, they can promote equality and respect, and they can facilitate companionship, comfort, and consensual sex. Men's lack of meaningful activity is a danger to the mental and emotional health of both men and women. Organizing and contributing to social activities and events can provide work as well as entertainment.

Questions about talents and skills might be added to surveys to identify those who can sing, draw, sew, or play sports, or who have organizational skills. Activities such as choirs, drama, or dance could be supported. Singing groups can involve both sexes, and provide an opportunity for pleasure and expression of

---

20. "Reproductive Health in Refugee Situations: Inter-Agency Field Manual," 1999. *www.rhrc.org/fieldtools/index.htm.*

21. W. Holmes, "HIV and Human Rights in Refugee Settings," *Lancet* 358 (2001): 144–46.

KEY INTERVENTIONS:
PREVENTING SEXUAL VIOLENCE

- Ensure that women have proper personal documentation for collecting food rations or shelter material.

- Increase availability of female protection officers and interpreters and ensure that all officers have knowledge of UNHCR Protection Guidelines and UN Security Guidelines for Women.

- Facilitate the use of existing women's groups or promote the formation of women's groups to discuss and respond to issues of sexual violence.

- Improve camp design for increased security for women.

- Include women in camp decision-making processes, especially in the areas of health, sanitation, reproductive health, food distribution, camp design/location.

- Distribute essential items such as food, water, and fuel directly to women.

- Train people at all levels (NGO, government, refugee, etc.), to prevent, identify, and respond to acts of sexual violence.

KEY INTERVENTIONS:
RESPONDING TO SEXUAL VIOLENCE

- Adapt WHO protocols to limit further traumas to survivors of sexual violence.

- Engage socially and culturally appropriate support personnel as a first contact with people who have been subjected to sexual violence.

- Provide prompt and culturally appropriate psychosocial support for survivors and their families.

- Provide medical follow-up immediately after an attack that also addresses STIs, HIV, infection and unwanted pregnancy.

- Establish closer links among protection officers, women's groups, traditional birth attendants, and community leaders to discuss issues related to the attacks.

- Document cases while respecting survivors' wishes and confidentiality.

⚘ DISCUSSION POINT ⚘

What advice can we give to women who have just been raped and are worried about the risk of HIV?

This is a sensitive question. Many women keep quiet about a rape because they feel ashamed or too upset to talk about it. Some women worry that they might not be believed or even that they might be blamed. It is good if a woman can tell a trusted family member or friend and ask that person to go with her to the police to report the rape. If the woman has access to health care services, she should go there as soon as possible so that she can be examined and so that samples can be taken that could help her if there is a court case against the perpetrator. Of course, women who have been raped want to wash as quickly as they can, but if they can receive a medical examination it is best to wait until after samples have been taken. In the protocols outlined in the WHO publications *Clinical Management of Survivors of Rape,* women are given the option of emergency contraception if they present within seventy-two hours of the rape, and the option of an IUD if they present within three to five days.

In some places emergency treatment with anti-HIV drugs might be available to try to prevent HIV infection.* Because the treatment remains unproven and can have side effects this should only be used when the risk of HIV infection is high. The treatment can be started soon after the rape, and the woman is likely to be able to take the drugs regularly for four weeks. It should not be used routinely and should never be considered a form of primary prevention.

Sometimes people ask whether a woman should wash out her vagina using a mild acid such as a vinegar or lemon juice solution, or even a cola drink, after a rape. It is true that HIV is inactivated by milk acids, but unfortunately studies in monkeys show that HIV passes rapidly through the mucosa (skin) lining the vagina into the cells of the body.** This means that washing out the vagina after rape will not be effective in preventing infection. Washing the vagina also removes the evidence that the woman has been raped. We know that repeated or regular vaginal douching increases the risk of infection with HIV through sex.

*CDC, "Management of Possible Sexual, Injecting-Drug-Use, or Other Nonoccupational Exposure to HIV, Including Considerations Related to Antiretroviral Therapy," *Morbidity and Mortality Weekly Report* 47 (1998): RR-17 2. I. M. Foster and J. Bartlett, "Anti-HIV Substances for Rape Victims," *Journal of the American Medical Association* 261 (1989): 3407.

**J. Hu, M. B. Gardner, and C. J. Miller, "Simian Immunodeficiency Virus Rapidly Penetrates the Cervicovaginal Mucosa after Intravaginal Inoculation and Infects Intraepithelian Dendritic Cells," *Journal of Virology* 74 (July 2000): 6087–95.

emotions, while performances provide much-needed entertainment. An enthusiastic sports trainer can help to motivate youth and provide a safe place for them to meet. These types of activities depend on identifying motivated leaders, and the main constraint is likely to be space.

Provide social activities for youth

Programs for youth are particularly important. Armed conflict often leaves a population with a disproportionate number of youth who are vulnerable to exploitation and have few skills or employment prospects. Often young people have to take on burdensome responsibilities for siblings or elderly relatives. Young people, especially girls, are at high risk of HIV, other STIs, unwanted pregnancy, and the complications of induced abortion.

Involve young people in their own needs assessment, which includes both the needs of unaccompanied young people and of youth-headed households. PLA methods are useful for this (see appendix C, page 201 for some ideas). Youth who are looking after young siblings may not be able to participate in school or youth center activities unless childcare can be arranged. There is a range of potential activities in refugee/IDP settings that could provide a sense of purpose and self-esteem for young people. It is important for young people to gain experience and skills that provide feelings of competence, self-respect, and hope that they will be able to make a living in the future. Meaningful activity and a sense of belonging to their community provide a counter to the factors that make young people likely to participate in high-risk behaviors.

Try to identify leaders among young people and give them recognition and acknowledgment. With a small amount of resources and some adult guidance young people might be encouraged to become involved in activities such as:

- setting up an open air "gymnasium,"
- looking after and teaching small children,
- learning traditional crafts from older people,
- organizing sports tournaments,

- forming music groups and planning entertainments,
- participating in protecting single women.

Provide community communication activities to change attitudes

Structured community discussions provide opportunities for men and women to better understand each other's perspectives and problems and have been found to be effective in altering HIV risk behaviors.

In 1995 a British NGO, ActionAid, produced the Stepping Stones training package, which helps communities to develop communication and relationship skills.[22] The package was designed for use in sub-Saharan Africa, but it has also been successfully adapted for use in Asia, North and Latin America, and Europe. It includes a manual for trainers and an accompanying workshop video. The package aims to enable individuals, their peers, and their communities to change their behavior — individually and together — through the "stepping stones" that the various sessions provide. Evaluations suggest that one of the most useful features of the Stepping Stones process is that the participants are divided into four small groups of ten to twenty, by age and gender: older men, older women, younger women, and younger men. All the groups are brought together for occasional sessions.

The aim of Stepping Stones is to enable women and men to describe and analyze their relationships and experiences and to develop solutions to the sexual health problems and risks that they face in the course of their daily lives. The materials enable people to explore issues that affect sexual health including gender roles, money, alcohol use, traditional practices, and attitudes to sex and death.

Stepping Stones is based on the following important principles:

- The best behavior change strategies are those developed by the members of a community themselves.

---

22. A. Welbourn, *Stepping Stones: A Training Package on HIV/AIDS, Gender Issues, Communication, and Relationship Skills* (London: ActionAid, 1995), *www.actionaid.org.*

PROMOTING UNITY:
A YOUTH PARTICIPATORY DEVELOPMENT PROGRAM

In Rwanda the IRC team has developed a Youth Participatory Development Program, in partnership with the Ministry of Youth, Sports, and Culture, to accomplish three primary objectives:

- to increase young people's capacity for participatory development by training democratically elected youth committees as a means of underscoring principles of coexistence and reconciliation,

- to ensure inclusion of all community youth in identifying problems and devising their own solutions by conducting participatory awareness campaigns in villages,

- to assist youth in planning and implementing viable, sustainable projects that promote their development through cooperative efforts that are inclusive of all community members.

During 1998, IRC conducted a youth-focused community planning exercise in Kibungo. Using PRA techniques, IRC was able to identify issues and needs of importance to youth. Using these findings as a framework, during 1999 IRC commenced a youth development program in two communes of Kibungo district, Birenga and Rutonde.

The expected outcomes include model programs to encourage youth participation, responsibility, and accountability; youth involved in their own development and civic society; increased productivity and cohesion through social, economic, and cultural activities; the promotion of marginalized and female youth through targeted participation; and improved reproductive health through peer education and counseling.

Thousands of youth have participated in assessment and planning sessions, in sports competitions, and in poetry and theater competitions with themes of peace, reconciliation, and HIV/AIDS.

- Peer groups need their own private time and space to identify and explore their own needs and concerns.

- The process of self-analysis leads to greater self-awareness and self-respect, and this enables people to practice more assertive behavior.

- The expression of our own needs leads to awareness of the needs of others, respect for others, better communication, and care.

- Behavior change will be more effective and sustained when the whole community is involved.

The sessions use a participatory approach of adult learning through shared discussions. The exercises are all based on people's own experiences. Role-play, drawing, and songs enable everyone to take part. Literacy is not required. Participants discuss their experiences, act them out, analyze them, consider alternative outcomes, and then rehearse these together in a safe, supportive group. This approach may also be helpful in challenging cultural practices that increase risk of the spread of HIV such as "widow cleansing," in which a dead man's brother has sex with his widow.

In some communities workshop sessions have been organized on a weekly basis, so four or five months are needed to complete the course. In other communities sessions have been held every afternoon five or six days a week, so that the course is completed in only three weeks. In some humanitarian settings it may be possible to conduct the sessions in this more intensive way. It may be difficult to get refugees or IDPs to engage in a process that they know is planned to take many months when they are hoping to go home as soon as possible, or when they are feeling fatalistic about the future.

It is important to bear in mind that in the safe environment created in the peer group sessions people may say more than they usually would. When these things are shared with the other groups the person may feel ashamed or embarrassed. Sometimes a woman may say something in a community meeting that gets her into trouble when she is alone with her husband. It is important that facilitators are well trained. In several countries the Stepping Stones process has resulted in greater openness and reduced stigma and fear.[23]

Support microfinance programs and income-generating activities

Poverty is the major reason for vulnerability to HIV infection. Refugees and IDPs are almost always poor and have generally lost their means of earning an income. In camp settings all their needs may be provided for, but in many settings refugees/IDPs try in a variety of ways to generate an income.

The United Nations Development Programme (UNDP) is interested in the possibilities for linking NGOs that try to respond to the HIV epidemic with microfinance institutions.[24] They point out that these institutions work at the community level, with poor people, predominantly women, and often hold weekly meetings with small groups. Information could be shared at these meetings. Partnerships between these types of organizations could have obvious benefits.

It is difficult, but not impossible, for NGOs to implement income-generating programs supported by small revolving loans. There have been many failures, and it is important to learn from these. Features that have been found to improve the chances of success include:

- consultation with local community structures;

- guidelines for management of the loan program with appropriate criteria for selection of beneficiaries and a clear policy for defaulters;

- small standardized loans with increased loan size available if the previous loan is repaid;

- realistic interest rates that cover management costs;

- individuals rather than groups, responsible for loans;

- training in budgeting, loan management, and skills associated with provision of loans;

- careful selection of appropriate activities for income generation, based on familiar and manageable activities such as selling vegetables or raising chickens, chosen by the beneficiary.

It is important to avoid providing loans to the indebted families who are too poor to repay a new debt. It is better to establish a savings plan or provide animals or food directly to the poorest families to avoid increasing their stress.

Income-generation activities can be designed to encourage women to be involved in a support group and community activities.

SUGGESTED INDICATORS

Clinic reports are not a reliable way to measure a decrease in STIs or incidents of sexual

---

23. N. Kaleeba et al., "Open Secret: People Facing Up to HIV and AIDS in Uganda," *Strategies for Hope Series 15*, *www.stratshope.org*.

24. UNDP, "Microfinance and HIV/AIDS: A Consultation on Joint Involvement in Effective Responses to HIV and AIDS," September 15–18, 1999.

violence in a population. This is because trends in these reports will depend on:

- quality of and access to services,

- awareness of the population,

- willingness to attend with an STI or after being raped,

- the quality of recording of consultations, as well as

- the actual rate of incidents of sexual violence or STI in the community.

Since any program that addresses these issues would hope to increase the quality and accessibility of services, raise awareness in the community, and improve reporting, as well as prevent the problems, we would expect rates of reported cases of STIs and sexual violence to increase initially. It is important to document reported rates of STIs and sexual violence, but such statistics need to be interpreted cautiously and in the light of other information from focus group discussions and community-based surveys.

PROVISION OF SERVICES

Indicator	Method of measurement
VCT services	
Proportion of population aware of VCT service by age and sex	Community survey
Numbers attending VCT service by age and sex	Review of records
Quality control system established for HIV tests	Observation, review of documents
Promotion and distribution of condoms	
Number of outlets distributing condoms	Observation, review of documents
Knowledge of correct condom use	Survey
Number of condoms distributed per month per capita	Distribution records
Increase in use of condoms with last sexual intercourse (with regular partner or with nonregular partner), among specified groups	Survey among specified groups
Change in attitudes toward condoms	Focus group discussions
Prevention and management of STIs	
Increase in knowledge of men and women in relation to STIs	Survey
Improved quality of documentation of consultations for STIs at the clinic	Focus group discussions Review of clinic records
Proportion of patients with an STI appropriately managed according to the syndromic management protocol	Clinic observation checklist
Proportion of STI patients who receive condoms by age and sex	Review of clinic records
Number of health workers trained in syndromic management of STIs	Review of training reports
Increased satisfaction of men and women with treatment for STIs	Focus group discussions
Reduction in prevalence of STIs among pregnant women	Survey of prenatal clinic attenders (with genital examination and swabs or urine specimens for PCR testing if available)

CHANGING INDIVIDUAL BEHAVIORS: INFORMATION, EDUCATION, AND COMMUNICATION

IEC Materials

Numbers and range of IEC materials produced as planned to support interventions	Review of materials
Numbers of IEC materials distributed appropriately	Observation Community survey
Target groups reached and messages understood	Focus group discussions Community survey
Changed attitudes, beliefs, and knowledge	Focus group discussions Community survey

SOCIETAL CONTEXT

Prevent sexual violence and provide care for survivors

Increased feeling of safety among women and young people	Survey Focus group discussion
Protocols available for psychosocial and medical care of survivors of sexual violence	Observation Review of protocols
Proportion of survivors of sexual violence who receive appropriate psychosocial and medical care within a specified time period	Clinic records
Number of health/social workers trained to manage survivors of sexual violence	Review of training reports
Increased awareness that care and counseling are available for survivors of sexual violence	Survey Focus group discussions
Proportion of reports of sexual violence that result in a penalty for the perpetrator	Will depend on circumstances — definition of "penalty," etc.
Changes in attitudes and practices as described by different groups within the community	Participatory processes

ADDITIONAL RESOURCES

General

"The Reproductive Health of Refugees." Special supplement. Ed. Laurel Shreck. *International Family Planning Perspectives* 26 (2000): 161–92.

UNAIDS. *Acting Early to Prevent AIDS: The Case of Senegal.* UNAIDS Best Practice Collection, 1999.

Voluntary counseling and testing

UNAIDS. *The Importance of Simple Rapid Assays in HIV Testing.* HIV VCT Evaluation Guides. *www.unaids.org.*

UNAIDS/WHO. *Guidelines for Using HIV Testing Technologies in Surveillance.* Geneva: UNAIDS/WHO Working Group on Global HIV/AIDS/STI Surveillance, 2001.

Condoms

Gardner, R., R. D. Blackburn, and U. D. Upadhyay. "Closing the Condom Gap." Population Reports, Series H, no. 9. Baltimore: Johns Hopkins University School of Public Health, Population Information Program, April 1999. Available at *www.jhuccp.org.*

"Reproductive Health: New Perspectives on Men's Participation." Population Reports, Series J, no. 46. Baltimore: Johns Hopkins University School of Public Health, Population Information Program, October 1998.

STI management and control

Adler, M., et al. *Sexual Health and Care: Sexually Transmitted Infections — Guidelines for Prevention and Treatment.* London: Overseas Development Administration, 1996. £6.95. Copies can be obtained, free of charge, by people working in developing countries from International Family Health, 13 Northburg St., London EC1V 0AH (tel.: 0171-336-6677; fax: 0171-336-6688; e-mail: *IFH-UK@dial.pipex.com*).

Dallabetta, G., M. Laga, and P. Lamptey. *Control of Sexually Transmitted Diseases: A Handbook for the Design and Management of Programs.* AIDSCAP/Family Health International, 1997.

UNAIDS. *The Public Health Approach to STD Control.* UNAIDS Technical Update. May 1998.

WHO. *Management of Patients with Sexually Transmitted Diseases.* WHO Technical Series Report Series 810, 1991.

WHO Initiative on HIV/AIDS and Sexually Transmitted Infections (HSI). *STD Case Management Course. www.who.int/.*

WHO/UNAIDS. *Sexually Transmitted Diseases: Policies and Principles for Prevention and Care.* Geneva: WHO/UNAIDS, 1997.

Behavior change and communication

Behavior Change Communication Handbook Series. Arlington, Va.: AIDSCAP/Family Health International, 1996. Published in English, French, and Spanish. Available at *www.fhi.org* or from the Publications Coordinator, Family Health International, P.O. Box 13950, Research Triangle Park, NC 27709, USA. Free to workers in developing countries.

Nutbeam, D., and E. Harris. *Theory in a Nutshell: A Practitioner's Guide to Commonly Used Theories and Models in Health Promotion.* Sydney, Australia: National Centre for Health Promotion, 1998.

Parnell, B., and K. Benton. *Facilitating Sustainable Behavior Change: A Guidebook for Designing HIV Programs.* Melbourne: Macfarlane Burnet Institute for Medical Research and Public Health, 1999.

Starrs, A., and R. Rizzuto. *Getting the Message Out: Designing an Information Campaign on Women's Health.* New York: Family Care International, 1995. US$6.00/copy for recipients in Europe and North America and representatives of international organizations. 1 copy free; 2+ US$3.00/copy for recipients in developing countries. Order from Family Care International, 588 Broadway, Suite 503, New York, NY 10012, USA. *www.familycareintl.org.*

Tabbutt, J. *Strengthening Communication Skills for Women's Health: A Training Guide.* New York: Family Care International, 1995. Order from Family Care International, 588 Broadway, Suite 503, New York, NY 10012, USA. *www.familycareintl.org.*

UNAIDS. *Radio and HIV/AIDS: Making a Difference.* A guide for radio practitioners, health workers, and donors, by Gordon Adam and Nicola Harford. Media Action International UNAIDS Best Practice Collection Key Material.

Youth

Gordon, G. *Choices: A Guide for Young People.* Macmillan/TALC. 1999. Available at *www.unicef.org/ pubsgen/youngpeople-hivaids/index.html*

UNICEF. *Adolescence: A Time That Matters.* UNICEF 2002. Available on the Internet at *www.unicef.org/ pubsgen/youngpeople-hivaids/index.html.*

———. Fact Sheet. HIV/AIDS and Children Affected by Armed Conflict. Available at *www.unicef.org/ pubsgen/youngpeople-hivaids/index.html.*

———. Fact Sheet. Young People and HIV/AIDS. 2002. Available on the Internet at *www.unicef.org/pubsgen/ youngpeople-hivaids/index.html.*

———. *Young People and HIV/AIDS: Opportunity in Crisis*, July 2002. Available at *www.unicef.org/ pubsgen/youngpeople-hivaids/index.html.*

Watson, C., and Brazier E. *You, Your Life, Your Dreams: A Book for Adolescents.* Family Care International, and Straight Talk Foundation in collaboration with Deutsche Stiftung Weltbevölkerung, 2000. An information handbook designed for young people, aged fourteen to nineteen, to read themselves. An excellent resource for youth centers, schools, health facilities, libraries, and programs that serve young people in Anglophone Africa. US$12.00/copy for recipients in Europe and North America and representatives of international organizations. 1 copy free, 2+ US$6.00/copy for recipients in developing countries. Available at *www.familycareintl.org.*

Prevention and management of the consequences of sexual violence and coerced sex

Heise, L., M. Allsberg, and M. Gottemoeller. "Ending Violence against Women." Population Reports. August 2000, Series L, no. 11. Baltimore: Johns Hopkins University School of Public Health, Population Information Program, 1999.

Security Guidelines for Women, United Nations Security Coordination Office. New York: United Nations, 1995.

Sexual Violence against Refugees: Guidelines on Prevention and Response. Geneva: UNHCR, 1995.

UNHCR. *How To Guide: Community-based Response to Sexual Violence: Crisis Intervention Teams — Ngara, Tanzania.* Geneva: UNHCR, 1997.

———. UNHCR. *How To Guide: Developing a Team Approach to Prevention and Response to Sexual Violence — Kigoma, Tanzania.* Geneva: UNHCR, 1998.

WHO. *Emergency Contraception: A Guide for Service Delivery.* Geneva: WHO, 1998.

WHO/UNHCR. *Mental Health for Refugees.* Geneva: WHO/UNHCR, 1994.

9

Strategies for Prevention of Transmission through Injecting Drug Use

HIV spreads very easily between people who inject drugs together and share needles, syringes, and other injecting equipment. Blood drawn back into the syringe can pass directly into the bloodstream of the next person to use the syringe.

Because it is illegal to inject drugs, it is often difficult for governments and communities to admit openly that it occurs. Those who inject are often reluctant to admit their drug use or to seek information and treatment. This means that it is difficult to ask about the extent and nature of injecting drug use.

There are now an estimated 5.5 million people who inject drugs in the world. Since it is a hidden problem, there may be many more. There are people who inject in at least 128 countries.[1] Injecting drug use is spreading to Eastern Europe, Latin America, and, more recently, to African countries. Epidemics of HIV follow the spread of injecting drug use. Injecting drug use is the most common cause of transmission of HIV in many Asian countries (including Malaysia, Vietnam, Yunan province in China, and the northeastern states of India), parts of eastern Europe, several of the newly independent States, a number of Latin American countries, and some western European countries such as Spain and Italy. In the Russian Federation, more than half the reported HIV cases to date have been in injecting drug users.

The problem of injecting drug use does not occur in all humanitarian settings, but there are a number of reasons why it may be a major problem. Breakdown in law and order in chaotic situations allows organized criminals to traffic in drugs as well as people. Armed conflicts are linked with arms sales, and arms sales are often linked with drug production and trafficking. Refugees and IDPs in camp settings may be bored and fatalistic about the future. Drugs can provide excitement and an escape from the painful reality of life in a camp. Groups who inject together provide a ritual and a sense of belonging that is attractive to young people, especially to those who have lost their families. Taking drugs can relieve feelings of fear, anxiety, and depression and provide a way of coping with painful memories.

Military personnel may introduce new drugs, or new ways of taking drugs, to a displaced or conflict-affected population. As a result of mass displacements there may be a mixing of populations with different drug-taking behaviors.

Drugs that are commonly injected include:

- **Opiates** produced from opium, collected from the sap of the seedpods of the poppy plant. Opium contains morphine, which can be converted to heroin by a simple chemical process. There are also synthetic opiates such as methadone and pethidine. These substances share the ability to relieve pain and produce a detached and pleasant mood. They induce physical dependence leading to distressing withdrawal symptoms when the drug is stopped.

- **Stimulants** including cocaine from the coca leaf. These produce a sense of exhilaration and decrease fatigue and hunger. There are also synthetic stimulants such as amphetamines. These substances have a high potential for dependence and can lead to psychosis.

---

1. "Drug Use and HIV/AIDS UNAIDS Statement," United Nations General Assembly Special Session on Drugs, UNAIDS Best Practice Collection Key Material (Geneva: UNAIDS, 1999).

123

- **Depressants** including barbiturates and sleeping pills. These substances cause drowsiness or pleasant relaxation. They also lead to physical and psychological dependence.

Of course drugs that are legal in many countries — alcohol and tobacco — also have serious health consequences, but they are not injected and do not lead directly to the spread of HIV, so we do not discuss them here.

RATIONALE

It is usually difficult to get people to stop injecting drugs. However, many people who inject drugs do eventually stop. The idea of harm reduction is to reduce the harmful effects of injecting drugs for injecting drug users, their families, and their communities, until they cease injecting. The harmful effects of injecting drug use include:

- death from overdose,
- infection with blood-borne viruses including HIV, hepatitis B, and hepatitis C,
- spread of HIV or hepatitis B to sexual partners,
- abscesses and bacterial blood infections from dirty needles,
- embolism from impurities in the drug,
- family conflict,
- STIs and sexual violence associated with prostitution,
- crime and time in prison.

To prevent harm from drug use we need to work in three areas:

1. preventing people from starting to inject,
2. protecting the health of those who inject and their families,
3. providing support and treatment services to people who use and want to stop.

It can take a long time to prevent people from starting to use drugs, or to provide treatment and rehabilitation services to help people to stop using. However, it is possible to implement strategies to protect the health of those

who inject and their families more quickly, and it is important to do so because HIV spreads very rapidly among people who inject.

There is evidence that programs that supply sterile needles and injecting equipment are able to reduce the extent of spread of HIV among people who inject. A study in over eighty cities showed that the incidence of HIV decreased by 5.8 percent per year in the twenty-nine cities with needle-syringe programs (NSPs) and increased by 5.9 percent per year in those without.[2] Countries that implemented harm reduction strategies early in the HIV epidemic, such as Australia, New Zealand, the United Kingdom, the Netherlands, and Denmark, have had a much lower rate of infection among drug users than in other countries. There is a great deal of evidence that NSPs do not lead to increased drug use or the recruitment of new injecting drug users. NSPs also allow an opportunity to provide information and referral to treatment and rehabilitation services for those who want to stop injecting.

In settings where needles and syringes are difficult to obtain, the drug dealer often provides the injection as well as the drug. This inevitably leads to spread of blood-borne viruses as many people are injected with the same equipment. Sometimes drug users make and use their own substitutes for needles and syringes, including eyedroppers and plastic pen parts.

STRATEGIES

Strategies in each area need to be integrated. The detail of the interventions will depend on the situation analysis (see chapter 5). The first priority is to provide access to sterile needles and syringes. Experience in many countries shows that it is essential to involve those who inject, their families, and the community in planning and implementation.

Prevent people from starting to inject — for example:

- provide opportunities for a drug-free lifestyle (sports; skills training; art; music; jobs);

2. S. Hurley, D. J. Jolley, and J. M. Kaldor, "Effectiveness of Needle-Exchange Programmes for Prevention of HIV Infection," *Lancet* 349 (1997): 1797–1800.

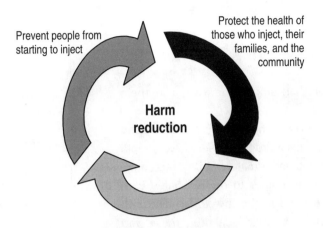

Prevent people from starting to inject

Protect the health of those who inject, their families, and the community

Harm reduction

Provide support and treatment services to those who want to stop injecting

Harm Reduction

- provide accurate information about drugs;

- educate police, teachers, and health and welfare professionals;

- strengthen a sense of community belonging and reconciliation;

- strengthen mental health services;

- strengthen opportunities for autonomy;

- foster sense of control;

- provide informal counseling services for young people;

- provide a place for young people to meet.

Protect the health of those who inject and their families:

- improve access to sterile needles, syringes, and injecting equipment; if it is necessary to re-use injecting equipment drug users need to know how to sterilize it through boiling or use of bleach between each use;

- inform those who inject and their families about blood-borne viruses;

- provide information about safer injecting practices;

- provide information about the danger of overdose and side effects of drugs;

- promote condom use;

- train health workers to manage overdoses and drug side effects;

- encourage those who inject to dispose of needles and syringes with care;

- improve access to health care services — reduce stigma and discrimination;

- provide informal counseling and support services to families;

- establish outreach education and peer education;

- encourage voluntary counseling and testing for HIV for those who inject drugs;

- advocate policy and legislative support for harm reduction strategies.

Provide support and treatment services to people who use and want to stop:

- provide opportunities for self-help groups and mutual support;

- train health workers and doctors in counseling, withdrawal strategies, drug substitution, and referral services;

- enable access to drug substitute programs;

- establish referral mechanism for residential detoxification services;

- provide support for home detoxification — including support and information for families.

Education and communication

The most effective way to reach those who inject is through outreach and peer education. Outreach workers are trained people from outside the community of injectors, although they may be former injectors. Peer educators are drug injectors trained to work with their community. IEC materials that seek to communicate with drug users need to be prepared by drug users because they understand what drug injectors do and why they do it. They can express messages in ways that other drug users will understand, and they have more credibility with drug users than health or prison officials.

Peer educators may undertake a range of tasks, including the provision of injecting equipment and bleach, the collection of used injecting equipment, and the dissemination of information about how to use bleach and issues related to health care and counseling.

⚑ DISCUSSION POINT ⚑

Why do people inject drugs rather than smoke them or take them by mouth?

It can be difficult for people who do not inject drugs to understand why people inject. When someone injects a drug the effect is very rapid because the drug enters the blood stream immediately. Drug users sometimes call this the "rush." Injecting soon comes to be associated with feeling the "rush." Needles are associated in the injector's mind with pleasure rather than pain. If they cannot get their usual drug, those who are used to injecting a drug will often inject some other drug, or even a substance that is not a drug.

When a drug becomes more expensive people are more likely to inject because they get more effect from the same amount of drug than if they smoke it or take it by mouth.

Injecting drug users often dissolve heroin in water and lemon juice in a spoon or bottle top over a candle; they may use cotton wool or cigarette filter tips as a filter when they draw up the drug. They use a tourniquet to enlarge their veins to make it easier to place the needle in the vein. Users often inject with others. The ritual of preparing a "fix" of their drug becomes important to those who inject. When they stop injecting, they miss the ritual, the companionship, and the rush of injecting, as well as the effects of the drug itself. Sharing any of this drug-injecting equipment, not just needles and syringes, carries a risk of transmission of HIV, hepatitis C, and hepatitis B.

Heroin users may inject two or three times a day, but cocaine users inject much more frequently because cocaine breaks down in the body more rapidly. It is almost impossible to supply sufficient needles and syringes to ensure that cocaine users inject safely.

If it is feasible to assist in setting up groups of people who inject drugs, they can be very effective at coordinating and supporting peer educators. However, the existence of such groups requires the cooperation of the police or law enforcement officers.

Advocacy and stigma reduction

The harm reduction approach is often controversial because it may be interpreted as condoning drug use. Advocacy is necessary; presenting harm reduction in a broad way that incorporates strategies to prevent drug use can help. It is unfortunate that debates about how to prevent harm from drug use are sometimes presented as two extreme positions: an approach of "zero tolerance" toward drug use, in which drug use becomes a stigmatized, secret, and hidden activity, and, on the other hand, encouragement of drug use by giving users the equipment they need to inject. In fact there is evidence that a harm reduction approach does not lead to increased use of drugs.

Injecting drug use is a heavily stigmatized behavior in most societies. There may be disapproval of the pleasure drug users obtain from their drug use, and understandable resentment of the crimes that drug users commit and their neglect of their families and responsibilities. As a result drug users become marginalized.

One way to reduce stigma associated with injecting drug use is to ensure that needles and syringes are not discarded in public spaces. Needles and syringes left in public spaces are a source of danger to others, especially children who may play with them. They cause great concern and anger. Campaigns to clear away needles and syringes and to ensure that they are properly and carefully disposed of can do much to reduce anger against drug users and NSPs.

If being in possession of injecting equipment is a crime, then those who inject are more likely to share needles and syringes. Education of police and advocacy with those who make and implement laws is necessary when planning an NSP. Local police may have a good understanding of the drug-using context and have often been willing to cooperate when they understand the benefits to the community as well as to the drug users.

Advocacy through peer education is likely to be most effective. Just as injecting drug users and others at risk of HIV are most likely to trust and believe their peers, so law-making officials, political and military leaders, and police officials are most likely to be persuaded by their peers.

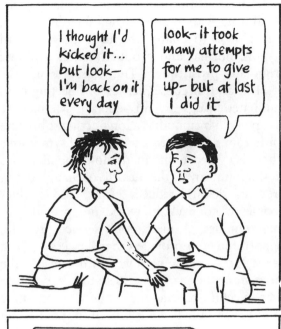

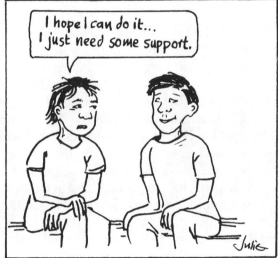

Needle-syringe programs

If injecting drug use is a problem in your setting, it is important to consider the establishment of an NSP. This may be situated in a health clinic or a welfare or youth center, or it may be run by outreach workers. The situation analysis should provide information about the most appropriate places to situate NSPs. Involve injecting drug users and the community in the planning. But be aware that this issue can be a source of much conflict in a community because people may worry that an NSP in their health center "normalizes" the use of drugs. Also, those who inject drugs may be reluctant

to visit health centers because they fear discrimination. Outreach workers need to be well trained, supervised, and supported.

Consult with injecting drug users to estimate the numbers of needles and syringes that will need to be ordered. Monitor the use closely so that sufficient supplies are in stock.

Drug treatment programs

It is possible to stop heroin use abruptly ("cold turkey"), but to do so is painful and causes symptoms of diarrhea and muscle pains as well as severe cravings for the drug. Relapse is common.

"Drug substitution" means replacing the usual drug with another drug taken by mouth. The aim is to enable the drug user to lead a more normal and productive life, avoiding crime and prostitution. The risks of overdose, of HIV, and of consequences of injecting contaminated drugs are all reduced. Methadone syrup taken by mouth is a long-acting substitute for heroin that prevents withdrawal symptoms. There is evidence that methadone maintenance is safe, improves the health of many users, prevents deaths, reduces crime, and enables people to go back to work and provide for their families. A methadone service provides opportunities to provide other services to drug users. However, some injectors do misuse the methadone they are prescribed: they may sell or even inject the methadone, while some continue to inject heroin. There is a need for counseling and support.

It will not be possible to establish drug substitution programs in unstable or temporary settings. An important principle of these programs is that the supply of methadone or other drug substitute needs to be consistent. If you are able to establish a methadone program for refugees or IDPs, try to ensure that the local host population also has access to the service.

Experience shows that if drug users wait for weeks to get into a treatment and rehabilitation program, by the time it is their turn they may have lost their motivation. Only voluntary detoxification is effective in the long term. When drug addictions are "treated" in prison or prison-like rehabilitation centers, relapse rates are high, especially when family members or the authorities arrange the detention.

Buprenorphine is a synthetic painkiller. When the price of heroin increases some drug users begin using buprenorphine as an alternative. In recent years it has been used successfully as a drug substitute for people who are dependent on opiates. In some countries it is cheaper and more readily available than methadone. Buprenorphine is a good substitute drug for people with low to moderate opiate dependency because it has few side effects and only mild withdrawal symptoms, and it does not need to be taken every day. A drop-in center can be established for clients to visit twice a week and receive health care and counseling support as well as buprenorphine.[3]

ADDITIONAL RESOURCES

Crofts, N., and D. Herkt. "A History of Peer-Based Drug User Groups in Australia," *Journal of Drug Issues* 25 (1995): 599–616.

Des Jarais, D. C. "Harm Reduction: A Framework for Incorporating Science into Drug Policy," *American Journal of Public Health* 85 (1995): 10–12.

Drucker, E. "Harm Reduction: A Public Health Strategy," *Current Issues in Public Health* (1995): 64–70. *www.lindesmith.org.*

Friedman, S., W. De Jong, and A. Wodak. "Community Development as a Response to HIV among Drug Injectors." *AIDS* Suppl. 1 (1993): S263–S269.

Manual for Reducing Drug Related Harm in Asia. The Centre for Harm Reduction, Macfarlane Burnet Institute for Medical Research and Public Health, and Asian Harm Reduction Network. Available at *www.chr.asn.au.*

UNAIDS. *Drug use and HIV/AIDS.* June 1998.

Wodak, A., N. Crofts, and R. Fisher. "HIV Infection among Injecting Drug Users in Asia: An Evolving Public Health Crisis," *AIDS Care* 5 (1993): 315–22.

---

3. J. Dorabjee, L. Samson, and R. Dyalchand, "A Community Based Intervention for Injecting Drug Users (IDUs) in the New Delhi Slums," WHO Drug Substitution Project Meeting on Opioid Substitution Programs in Asia, Kathmandu, February 1997.

HARM REDUCTION AMONG REFUGEES IN HONG KONG

Pillar Point in Hong Kong was opened as a transit camp for Vietnamese people awaiting departure to a country of asylum. The camp is in an area well known for drug use and criminal activity. The difficult conditions, sense of helplessness and hopelessness about the future, the pleasure and social acceptance of drugs among the male refugees have led to much heroin use in the camp. It is estimated that up to 95 percent of the men are dependent. They work mainly as day laborers and most now have criminal records, which block their chances of resettlement. In July 1996 Médecins Sans Frontières began a harm reduction program among drug users. Their aims were to reduce the health risks of injecting drugs and to improve the overall quality of the lives of those who inject and their families. They planned to raise awareness of the health-related risks, to encourage safer injecting practices and safer sex, to encourage safer disposal of used needles and syringes, and to help injectors gain access to methadone programs.

The field team was composed of a Vietnamese drug counselor and a doctor: they worked in the evening and on the weekends, as this was the best time to reach injecting drug users. The workers offered confidential individual counseling sessions at which alternatives of drug treatment and safer injecting practices would be discussed. They also gave out a pack containing three needles and syringes, three sterile water vials, three sterile swabs, one condom and a leaflet with appropriate information about STIs, HIV/AIDS, and condoms. They discussed methods of safer using and listened to concerns. Individual needle and syringe boxes, closed by a tamper-proof seal, were distributed and, when used, collected by the doctor. A three-month survey of the program's clients found that:

- 70 percent of injecting drug users had not shared needles and syringes;
- 30 percent of those who had shared had cleaned the needle and syringe before injecting;
- 81 percent always cleaned their skin with a swab before injecting;
- 74 percent used boiled or sterile water to mix up their drug.

They also found that 75 percent of their clients were concerned about disposal issues and understood the danger that discarded needles and syringes could be to other people, especially to the children in the camp. The camp has now become free of discarded needles and syringes.

—G. Nemayechi and T. Taveaux, "Médecins Sans Frontières HARP (Harm Reduction Program) for the Vietnamese Drug Users in Pillar Point Refugee Camp," July 1996–April 1997. Evaluation report in the *Manual for Reducing Drug Related Harm in Asia*. The Centre for Harm Reduction, Macfarlane Burnet Institute for Medical Research and Public Health and Asian Harm Reduction Network.

SUGGESTED INDICATORS

Indicator	*Method of measurement*
Plan to address risk of spread of HIV through injecting drug use developed with injecting drug users	Review of documented plan
Numbers of teachers, police, health, and welfare workers trained in harm reduction for injecting drug use issues	Training reports
Improved understanding of the harm reduction approach among key officials, teachers, police, health and welfare workers, and the general community	Focus group discussions and in-depth interviews
Centers or activities available for youth	Observation, camp documents
Injecting drug users aware of and able to access sterile needles and syringes	Interview survey
Number of needles and syringes exchanged or distributed	Needle-syringe exchange program records
Pre-tested information materials available about how to prevent spread of blood-borne viruses through injecting drug use	Review of materials
Public spaces free of discarded needles and syringes	Systematic observation
Number of peer educators trained	Review of training reports
Number of peer educator contacts	Review of logbooks of peer educators
Number of health workers trained	Review of training reports
Proportion of clients in drug substitution program that have been followed up appropriately	Clinic records
Proportion of clients that have relapsed and gone back to injecting drugs six months after completing the substitution program	Follow-up survey
Decreased HIV incidence among injecting drug users	Annual anonymous unlinked survey
Improved quality of life of drug users and their families	In-depth interviews and focus group discussions

10

Enabling People to Live Positively with HIV

HIV-positive people are often seen only in terms of being "victims" or "carriers" of a deadly virus. They are usually unable to discuss their status openly because of the stigma associated with AIDS. But increasingly people living with HIV/AIDS (PLWH/A)[1] are looking at life beyond diagnosis; HIV infection needs to be viewed as a chronic, long-term disease. With acceptance, good nutrition, and care and support, people with HIV live long and productive lives.

PLWH/A have much to contribute to the design, implementation, monitoring, and evaluation of HIV prevention and care activities. There is a strong link between the promotion of the rights of PLWH/A and prevention of the spread of HIV. PLWH/A often have much to tell about local treatment, care, and support services, including ideas on how they can be improved. Supporting PLWH/A to speak about their own experiences is a valuable behavior change strategy.

RATIONALE

What do we mean by "people living with HIV"?

Most people who are living with HIV do not know that they are infected. But some who have never had a test may suspect or believe that they have become infected with the virus, for example, the wife of a man who dies of an AIDS-related illness and who becomes sick with similar symptoms. Others may be quite unaware of the possibility of HIV infection. Among those who have tested positive for HIV, there are those who deny their HIV status, either consciously or subconsciously, and continue to believe that they are not infected.

Some of those who accept that they have HIV choose not to tell anyone. Some may tell their partner or closest friend; some tell most of their family and friends; others are willing to become publicly positive and to talk about living with HIV with people that they do not know. Some people are willing to become publicly positive soon after their diagnosis; some may take time to tell family and friends gradually before they start to talk in public. Others may be willing to talk to people that they do not know — but do not want to tell their family or their work colleagues, for a variety of reasons. It is important not to make assumptions and to respect the right of PLWH/A to choose who they want to tell. We should also remember that there are PLWH/A who did not choose to publicize their HIV status but because of a lapse of confidentiality it became public knowledge. When working with PLWH/A it is vital to maintain confidentiality.

Any of the above groups of PLWH/A may contribute to the field of HIV prevention and care, not only those who are willing or able to be publicly positive. In addition, it is vital to hear and consider the views of those who are affected by HIV — the family, friends, and lovers of those infected.

Much of this chapter has been adapted from the chapter "Positive Response: The Central Role of HIV+ People" by Susan Paxton in *Community Action on HIV: A Resource Manual for Prevention, Care and Support*, 2d ed., ed. Tamara Kwarteng, Rob Moodie, and Wendy Holmes (Melbourne: Macfarlane Burnet Institute for Medical Research and Public Health, September 2002).

1. Some people with HIV do not like the term "People living with HIV" because it might carry the suggestion that their infection status defines their life. However, the acronym PLWH (or PLWH/A) is widely used, including by groups of HIV-positive people, so we use it here as a convenient way to talk of people who are infected with HIV. It is important to note that different people are sensitive about different terms, and it is always useful to discuss these issues with those you work with.

Stigma

PLWH/A have the same rights to privacy, freedom from violence, freedom of movement, housing, employment, care and support, and access to health care as those who are not infected. Yet positive people are often deprived of their rights because of the stigma surrounding AIDS. People are often afraid to talk about AIDS because it means talking about culturally taboo subjects such as sex and death. So they push it away and convince themselves that HIV affects only particular groups, "other" people. They transfer their fears onto those already living with the virus.

We need to encourage people to talk openly about AIDS and listen to what HIV-positive people have to say about their experience. By creating an environment in which PLWH/A have a voice, people begin to identify with those living with the virus, and attitudes to AIDS begin to change. The issue of HIV becomes more familiar, and stigma and discrimination decrease. People begin to examine their own risk of infection in a responsible way.

The Paris AIDS Summit Declaration, signed by forty-two countries, states that the success of HIV prevention and care programs depends on the full participation of PLWH/A.[2] The Declaration commits governments to consult with affected groups, eliminate discrimination against PLWH/A, and decrease women's vulnerability to HIV. In order to carry out this commitment to greater involvement of PLWH/A, the declaration acknowledges the need to strengthen the skills of HIV-positive people.

HIV often robs people of control over their life. A positive diagnosis is accompanied by loss, disempowerment, and social ostracism. Rather than become victims many PLWH/A choose to respond in a positive way to their situation. Often they are passionately motivated to contribute to HIV prevention and care. If a strategy is in place to ensure adequate training and support, positive people can be involved at

every level of the community response to AIDS. They might become involved in:

- counseling, care, and support;

- disseminating information to others infected with HIV;

- prevention programs, including raising awareness and educating the community, or in working groups designing models of health care and service delivery.

Because of stigma there are few who are willing to make their positive HIV status public, so those who do have a huge burden of work, with little opportunity to gain support from each other. PLWH/A meeting in Kenya described four areas of stigma that need to be addressed:

1. **Self-stigmatization:** avoidance of people, withdrawal, depression, and self-hatred. This may be expressed as low self-esteem and playing the role of an ill person or "victim." This has a negative impact on mental well-being and in turn on physical health.

2. **Stigma from the health care sector:** apathy in medical services, judgmental attitudes from counselors, nursing, and medical staff, compulsory or involuntary disclosure, and denial of treatment or sterilization without informed consent.

3. **Stigma in representation and communication:** stigma due to careless language and unclear terminology used by the media, social leaders, and society in general. Stigma arises from misrepresentation of PLWH/A as people who are dying from, rather than living with, a virus. Misconceptions are also presented about the behavior of PLWH/A, particularly sexual behavior. Misinformation about routes of transmission of HIV generates discrimination and fear. Finally, tokenism is an additional source of stigma for PLWH/A, when individuals are used for the needs of other people or organizations.

4. **Social and work environments:** hostility, violence, silence, and denial about HIV/AIDS often leading to exclusion of PLWH/A. Environments include work, housing, and insurance

---

2. Declaration of the Paris AIDS Summit (Section IV, Paragraph 1) available at *www.unaids.org/whatsnew/conferences/summit/index.html.*

systems. The children of PLWH/A may be ostracized at school and in the community.[3]

STRATEGIES

Protect the human rights of people living with HIV/AIDS

Relief agencies can assist PLWH/A to document and describe the human rights issues they face and examine the impact of discrimination on their quality of life in order to achieve changes in attitudes, policy, and legislation. If possible they should be helped to contact other PLWH/A groups in the region or in other countries (see addresses below, page 218). For example, APN+, the Asia Pacific Network of People Living with HIV/AIDS, has undertaken a peer-based project to document violations of human rights in a systematic way and has found that the majority of people diagnosed with HIV experience discrimination within the health sector.

When IEC materials are produced in relation to any aspect of HIV care and prevention there is an opportunity to address stigma and ignorance. Materials can also be produced specifically to counter fear, stigma, and discrimination. PLWH/A may be invited to speak at important occasions such as the opening of a building, the launch of a new program, judging a competition, or meeting a visiting dignitary. Encourage representation of PLWH/A on refugee/IDP committees, hospital boards, and local government advisory committees.

Many health professionals do not learn about HIV during their original training and may be ignorant about the transmission and management of HIV infection. Because doctors and nurses tend to be trusted opinion leaders, health care consultations can be a potent generator of stigma, especially if other staff and patients observe the doctor taking unnecessary precautions. On the other hand consultations can provide an opportunity to reduce stigma and fear by demonstrating that physical contact does not transmit HIV and providing an example of compassion and respect. Health professionals need clear information about transmission routes and universal precautions (see page 170), as well as their obligations to respect the rights of PLWH/A. Invite PLWH/A to assist in planning and teaching training courses for health workers to improve the care health workers provide to people with PLWH/A and to explain their information needs.

Establish peer support groups

Because positive people are marginalized and isolated it is important to create a supportive environment in which they can contribute effectively. The first step is to facilitate peer support. This means enabling HIV-positive people to meet each other in a safe, comfortable, and confidential environment. Lack of space and fear of identification may make this difficult in refugee/IDP settings where there may be a lack of trust. In insecure environments, fear and discrimination flourish. The prime purpose of support groups is to empower PLWH/A to live satisfying and productive lives. Members of support groups know that there will be someone to care for them when they are ill, just as they have cared for others.

"Peer support" may be as simple as two people having an opportunity to meet with each other. Once a group is established, other people will join. It is a good idea for the group members to decide some rules early on. Some examples are: "Listen to each other and respect what each other says." "Everything discussed in the group will stay in the group and will not be discussed with others outside the group." Peer groups can help PLWH/A to understand their own health and treatment information through newsletters and workshops. Contact details for the group can be given to PLWH/A during post-test counseling. Resources should be set aside for publicity. There is a particular need to attract men as members. Men are often more reluctant than women to acknowledge their positive status to themselves or others.

Build capacity and enhance skills of PLWH/A

Talk to positive people who want to offer their time. Find out about their skills and experience

---

3. "Report of the Technical Consultation on Greater Involvement of People Living with HIV/AIDS (GIPA)," March 2000, Nairobi, Kenya.

and what they would like to learn. This might include:

- basic facts about HIV and AIDS;
- advocacy, public speaking, and media skills;
- counseling;
- group development and facilitation skills, and meeting procedures;
- financial management;
- strategic planning and organizational skills;
- evaluation and monitoring;
- proposal writing;
- home-based care;
- stress management.

Acknowledge the skills and talents that refugees/IDPs who are positive already have. Positive people who have become actively involved in AIDS work include writers, nurses, performers, farmers, doctors, teachers, and lawyers.

Train counselors to give psychological support to PLWH/A

Because HIV-positive counselors often have an immediate understanding of many of the issues their clients face, they may be highly sought after. They can become overwhelmed by the many demands and need supportive counseling or spiritual guidance.

Many women living with HIV already care for partners and children who also have the virus; some PLWH/A are involved in home care programs. Those who carry this double load need additional care and support themselves. Being a home-based care volunteer can be satisfying but may also be emotionally overwhelming when it makes PLWH/A think about their own future. The death of a client can be a particularly difficult time for positive carers, and counseling should be available to them.

Make sure that positive volunteers involved with your organization have basic health care, including adequate shelter, a good diet, and

access to treatments for opportunistic infections. Maintaining the confidentiality of HIV-positive clients and volunteers is vital.

At times professionals may be reluctant to involve positive people. Often workers are so preoccupied with responding to the immediate demands placed on them that it is difficult to step back and plan a strategy which recognizes, accepts, and supports the participation of PLWH/A. It is important to be flexible and to collaborate with positive people as equal partners.

PLWH/A should never be pressured to disclose their infection as a service to the community. It is important to emphasize here that while the involvement of infected and affected people in HIV prevention efforts is encouraged, this should happen only in an environment where disclosure of their HIV-positive status will not endanger their lives or lead to discrimination.

Taking an active part in HIV programs can be one way that PLWH/A can regain a sense of control. It has enriched the lives of many, giving them dignity and self-respect. PLWH/A visibility is also inspiring for other positive people and helps them to develop a more optimistic outlook. They realize that it is possible to live a healthy, useful, and fulfilling life with HIV.

ADDITIONAL RESOURCES

"Enhancing the Greater Involvement of People Living with or Affected by HIV/AIDS in Sub-Saharan Africa." October 2000. *www.unaids.org/publications/documents/persons/index.html.*

Paxton, S. "The Impact of Utilizing HIV-Positive Speakers in AIDS Education," *AIDS Education and Prevention* 14 (2002): 282–94.

———. *Lifting the Burden of Secrecy: A Manual and Training Module for HIV-Positive People Who Want to Speak Out in Public.* Asia-Pacific Network of People Living with HIV/AIDS. Available at *www.hivasiapacific.apdip.net*

———. "The Paradox of Public HIV Disclosure," *AIDS Care* 14 (2002): 559–67.

SUGGESTED INDICATORS

Indicator	Method of measurement
Proportion of health care workers (of all levels) trained in nondiscriminatory care and their obligations toward human rights of PLWH/A	Training reports
Written information materials for health professionals to reduce stigma	Review of materials
Number of counselors trained in psychological support for PLWH/A	Training reports
Number of members of peer support groups for PLWH/A	Peer group reports
Details of support groups available at post-test counseling	Observation
Awareness of PLWH/A of peer support groups	Observation In-depth interviews
Testing for HIV always voluntary and accompanied by counseling	Review of VCT center records In-depth interviews with PLWH/A and staff
PLWH/A not segregated in clinics or hospital	Observation
Referral and follow-up mechanisms in place at VCT centers and peer support groups for other sources of care and support for PLWH/A	Observation Review of documents
Peer support groups functioning and accessible	In-depth interviews with PLWH/A and support group members

Part 4

ISSUES FOR
HEALTH CARE SERVICES

Although the response to the HIV epidemic needs to be intersectoral, there are some issues that are inevitably the concern of health care services, and they are dealt with in part 4. These issues include the prevention of the spread of the virus from parent to child (chapter 11), through blood transfusions (chapter 12), and within clinics and hospitals (chapter 13). The continuum of care needs to extend to home-based care, but since this is most likely to be coordinated by health care services we have included the issue of providing care, and looking after the carers, in chapter 14.

11

Prevention and Care in Relation to Parent-to-Child Transmission

The number of children infected with HIV is increasing rapidly in countries where HIV in adults has spread widely. Most women who become infected with HIV are in the reproductive age group. Since the beginning of the AIDS pandemic, an estimated five million infants have been infected with HIV. In many countries the gains made in child survival have been lost because of AIDS. The problem has been greatest in sub-Saharan Africa, but the number of babies infected with HIV in India and Southeast Asia is also increasing rapidly. We use the term "parent-to-child transmission" (PTCT) when talking of public health and policy aspects to acknowledge the role of the father in transmission of HIV from mother-to-child. We use the term "mother-to-child transmission" (MTCT) when referring to the risk of transmission from an infected woman to her baby.

HIV infection in children

The babies of HIV-positive mothers have a higher risk of low birth weight, prematurity, stillbirth, and perinatal mortality. The most common clinical features of HIV infection in children are:

- failure to thrive,
- recurrent bacterial infections, especially pneumonia,
- recurrent and persistent diarrhea,
- oral thrush (candidiasis),
- generalized enlargement of the lymph glands,
- itchy rashes,
- chronic cough,
- enlarged liver and spleen,
- developmental delay, and
- neurological problems.

Diagnosis of HIV infection in children is difficult before eighteen months of age because maternal HIV antibodies cross the placenta. Most of the signs and symptoms of HIV infection in children are common and nonspecific, which makes it difficult to be certain of a clinical diagnosis. Tuberculosis, malnutrition, persistent diarrhea, and congenital syphilis can all be confused with HIV. They can also all occur in HIV-infected children.

The course of HIV disease in most HIV-infected infants is more rapid than in adults. Children who develop manifestations of HIV infection before one year of age have a poor prognosis. Their condition usually deteriorates until they die within three years. Some children develop symptoms for the first time in their second or third year. Many of these children continue to grow well, although they may have frequent minor illnesses. These different patterns of progression may be explained by different viral strains, genetic factors in the host, the timing of infection, the immune status of the mother, and co-factors such as other infections.

Impacts of PTCT

Many women will first discover their HIV infection, and that of their husband, when their baby becomes ill. Women whose babies fail to thrive may be blamed by their husband or relatives. Most women do not know whether they are infected with HIV. As awareness of the possibility and consequences of PTCT increases, women may fear becoming pregnant. Pregnant women worried about HIV need supportive counseling and information about risks, including acknowledgment of areas of uncertainty,

139

and about actions that couples or women themselves can take to reduce the risk of PTCT. Once the baby is born, parents have to cope with uncertainty until the baby is old enough for diagnosis. Parents, especially mothers, of infected babies have to cope with the burden of recurrent illness of their child without hope of recovery. This often leads to many trips to clinic, hospital, or traditional healer, which cost money, take time, and cause distress. The burden can be managed more successfully at home if families have support, information, and access to simple medicines (see page 177). Responsibility for orphaned babies may mean that older girls cannot attend school, or that elderly people become exhausted, so respite care is needed. Forced migration with children is always difficult, but when a child has a chronic illness the burden on families is even greater.

Nurses, midwives, and health care professionals have to cope with uncertainty, rapidly changing knowledge, their own fears, and not being able to cure the disease. Dealing with the fears of women and their families, and with sick and dying children, is very stressful. It is easy for them to feel overwhelmed.

The uninfected children of infected parents have higher risk of illness than children of uninfected parents in the same settings and suffer the emotional and social effects of the chronic illness and death of their parents. Around the world, over eleven million children have already lost their mothers — and often their fathers — before they were fifteen years old. Some argue against efforts to prevent PTCT of HIV on the grounds that more children of HIV-infected mothers will survive to become orphans that need care. Clearly this is not an ethically defensible argument. Even with effective interventions in place there will still be many orphans, and children infected with HIV will require more costly care than if they were uninfected.

RATIONALE

By paying attention to the factors that increase the risk that HIV will pass from mother to child, there is much that can be done to prevent PTCT. You might want to reread the information about the risk and timing of transmission from mother to child and the influences on this risk presented on page 23.

The pace of change in our knowledge about interventions to prevent the spread of the virus to the baby from an infected mother has been rapid. It is difficult for policy makers to know what to recommend in poor but stable settings. It is even more difficult in humanitarian settings and during population displacement.

The interventions that can help prevent PTCT of HIV relate to areas of life that have great cultural and social significance — sexual behavior, the desire to have babies, pregnancy, childbirth, the postpartum period, and infant feeding. They are areas of intimate concern to women, yet often governed by men. They are also areas of life that are greatly affected when populations are displaced as a result of conflict.

Primary prevention

The best way to prevent babies becoming infected with HIV is primary prevention — that is, to prevent the spread of the virus between men and women (see parts 3 and 4). Community education to raise awareness that babies can be infected with HIV can contribute to primary prevention by appealing to men's sense of responsibility for their families.

To prevent PTCT it is particularly important to prevent women becoming infected with HIV during pregnancy, at delivery, or while lactating. This is because the peak in viral load that occurs in the weeks after infection means that the risk of transmission to the baby then is much higher than for a woman who has been infected for longer and has a low viral load. Husbands may become infected through unprotected sex outside marriage during pregnancy or the weeks after the birth. They will be particularly infectious due to a high viral load when marital sex is resumed. Increased vascularity of the woman's genitals during pregnancy and post-partum may increase her vulnerability to infection. It is also important to minimize blood transfusions during childbirth through training midwives in active management of third stage of labor and strict transfusion criteria (see page 161).

Secondary prevention

Secondary prevention means preventing transmission of HIV to the baby when the mother is infected. In recent years most attention has been given to secondary prevention interventions that depend on testing women for HIV during pregnancy: antiretroviral prophylaxis, avoidance or modification of breast-feeding, and elective caesarean section. But since the majority of infected pregnant women do not know their HIV status, it is also important to allocate resources to the secondary prevention strategies that do not depend on testing during pregnancy. Few women have access to prenatal VCT as yet, and those who do may prefer not to be tested for HIV, or may not be in a position to decide. The secondary prevention strategies that do not depend on testing also assist the health of women and men in general. These include:

- preventing unwanted pregnancies through increasing access to information and contraception;

- improving the health and nutrition of pregnant women and treating infections, especially STIs, promptly;

- promoting exclusive breast-feeding for all;

- providing breast-feeding training for health care workers to minimize breast problems;

- encouraging women with any chronic illness to postpone pregnancy;

- avoiding unnecessary obstetric interventions, especially artificial rupture of membranes.

Many of these activities may be components of existing reproductive health, or maternal and child health programs, but the recognition that they make an important contribution to the prevention of PTCT of HIV justifies investment of increased resources.

Test-dependent interventions

Antiretroviral prophylaxis

A short course of zidovudine (AZT) during the last four weeks of pregnancy and three hourly doses during labor reduce the risk of MTCT by half when babies are not breast fed. In breast-fed populations the efficacy of this regimen is reduced. This intervention has been implemented widely in Thailand saving many babies from HIV infection. However, Thailand is a middle-income country with a good health infrastructure and stable and cohesive communities. These interventions have proved more difficult to implement in poorer and less stable settings in Africa and Asia.[1]

A study in Uganda showed that a single dose of a different antiretroviral drug, nevirapine, given at the time of delivery to the mother, and then to the newborn, also reduces the risk of HIV infection by half. This intervention costs only a few dollars and is able to reduce the risk of transmission despite continued exposure to HIV during breast-feeding. WHO has approved nevirapine for widespread use, and this cheap and practical regimen is replacing zidovudine. The efficacy of antiretroviral prophylaxis (ARVP) given to the baby during the breast-feeding period is also being studied.

Common problems experienced in implementing prenatal VCT and ARVP include:

- providing training for sufficient clinic staff,

- the added workload of providing VCT in already overstretched clinics,

- lack of privacy for VCT,

- high rate of loss to follow-up of HIV-positive pregnant women, and

- low rates of take-up of antiretroviral prophylaxis.

If done well, the introduction of VCT at prenatal clinics can strengthen the quality of reproductive health services. If women who test negative, and their husbands, receive post-test counseling, prenatal VCT can contribute to primary prevention.

Elective caesarean section

Caesarean section before the onset of labor allows the baby to avoid contact with the

---

1. UNICEF, UNAIDS, WHO, UNFPA, "African Regional Meeting on Pilot Projects for the Prevention of Mother-to-Child Transmission of HIV," Gaborone, Botswana, March 27–31, 2000. *www.unaids.org.*

mother's blood and cervical secretions. Studies have shown that elective caesarean section for HIV-positive women can reduce the risk of PTCT by 50 to 66 percent. However, there is evidence that HIV-positive mothers have a higher risk of post-operative complications than HIV-negative women. In humanitarian settings it is important to consider the safety of caesarean section, the cost, whether women can access caesarean section surgery, and whether they will be able to do so for future pregnancies, since there will be an increased risk of rupture of the uterus with subsequent deliveries.

Modification of breast-feeding

For many years it was difficult for researchers to determine the size of the risk of transmission of HIV through breast-feeding. There is now sufficient evidence to show that nonexclusive breast-feeding carries a substantial additional risk of MTCT of HIV of between 10 and 16 percent. The risk is greatest in the early weeks, but remains throughout the duration of breast-feeding.

Breast-feeding plays a vital role in protecting children's health and has important nutritional and immunological benefits. Babies who are not breast fed have a high risk of death from malnutrition, diarrhea, and respiratory infections. Breast-feeding also has important child-spacing and psychological advantages. In humanitarian settings breast-feeding is even more important to child health because providing an adequate alternative requires supplies of milk, water, and fuel, which may be unavailable, and displaced populations may move again at short notice. If breast-feeding mothers have to move they have a safe, low-cost, sterile, convenient source of food for their baby.

The health benefits of breast-feeding are of most importance in the first six months of life, so shorter duration of breast-feeding by infected women may reduce risk of HIV transmission while allowing the benefits of breast-feeding in the early vulnerable months.

"Exclusive breast-feeding" means that the baby receives nothing but breast milk; it is a rare practice in all societies. It is common for water, sugar water, milk or herbal substances

to be given before the milk "comes in," and for cereals to be introduced in the first weeks of life. Breast milk contains both protective antibodies and growth factors that promote maturity of the intestinal wall. Babies do not need to receive any food or fluids other than breast milk for the first six months of life. Other fluids or foods result in inflammation of the intestinal wall that may increase the risk that HIV in the breast milk can enter the baby through the intestinal wall. The suggestion that exclusive breast-feeding may carry a lower risk of MTCT and even inhibit HIV transmitted to the baby at the time of delivery has been strengthened by findings from two observational studies.

Breast-fed babies need no food or drink other than their mother's milk until they are six months old. Babies fed on formula can start to have other foods from five or six months of age. Cereal porridge is fine as the first food for babies. At first they will still be getting most of their energy and growth needs from the milk they are drinking. When cereal porridge is cooked, a lot of water needs to be added to make sure that the porridge is not too sticky or thick for the baby to eat. This means that the porridge is energy dilute — or not very concentrated in energy. Babies and small children have small stomachs, so they need to be fed very often. There are several ways to add energy to porridge: (1) add milk, sugar, peanut butter, oil, margarine, ground fish, or eggs, (2) ferment the porridge, or (3) use germinated flour. Fermentation also reduces bacterial growth in porridge. It is also important to provide vitamins and minerals — in mashed bananas, and other fruit or vegetables. Mothers also need advice about the importance of hand washing before they prepare food for their baby, before they feed the baby, and after they clean the baby's bottom. They also need to learn to dispose carefully of the baby's stools. Children's stools are more dangerous than adult stools. It is best not to store cooked porridge or other foods for the baby. Instead mothers should give leftover food to other children or eat it themselves, rather than waste it. If possible prepare a pamphlet on safe weaning foods using information and pictures from the manual *Nutrition for Developing Countries.*[2]

There is an urgent need for further research to determine the safest pattern and duration of breast-feeding, and the feasibility and safety of alternatives to breast-feeding when they are needed.

The fact that breast-feeding carries a significant risk of transmitting a fatal infection presents policy makers with a genuine dilemma. The balance of risk will vary for different mothers in different settings.

In May 1998, WHO, UNICEF, and the Joint UN Programme on HIV/AIDS (UNAIDS) published new guidelines on infant feeding and HIV. The guidelines recommend that women known to be infected with HIV be counseled about the risks and, if feasible, helped to provide an adequate replacement for breast-feeding, even in poor countries. The guidelines stress the importance of protecting, promoting, and supporting breast-feeding as the best method of feeding for infants whose mothers are HIV-negative or who do not know their HIV status. These guidelines have recently been clarified:

HIV and infant feeding counseling in humanitarian settings

Balancing the risks

HIV-infected pregnant women need advice and counseling to help them to make an informed decision about whether to breast-feed or not.

Weighing the risks has been difficult in resource-poor settings because we know little about safe, feasible, and affordable alternatives to breast-feeding. In humanitarian settings exclusive breast-feeding for four to six months followed by early weaning is likely to be a much safer option for the baby than avoidance of all breast-feeding. It is true to say, currently, that we do not know which of these options carries a lower risk of HIV transmission to the baby, and avoidance of all breast-feeding is certainly hazardous.

2. F. Savage King and A. Burgess, *Nutrition for Developing Countries* (New York: Oxford University Press, 1993).

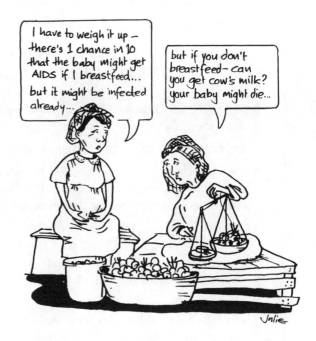

Promoting exclusive breast-feeding for all

Exclusive breast-feeding for six months should be strongly promoted and supported in refugee and IDP camps for all babies, both because it protects babies against diarrheal and other infectious diseases, and because it may reduce the risk of transmission of HIV from infected mothers. The ten steps to successful breast-feeding listed in the box on page 144 should be promoted in all hospitals or clinics where displaced mothers give birth.

Infant Feeding in Emergencies is a helpful book designed to give advice to refugee and internally displaced women about breast-feeding (see below page 158). The information can be adapted for women in your setting. Individual counseling about the benefits and practice of exclusive breast-feeding has been found to be more effective than just providing information. Counseling by someone trained in breast-feeding skills can help to reduce breast-feeding problems that increase risk, such as engorgement, mastitis, and sore nipples.

Replacement options

If an HIV-positive woman chooses not to breast-feed she will need support to provide an adequate replacement. Where few women are infected with HIV it may be possible for women who cannot afford infant formula

CURRENT RECOMMENDATIONS OF THE INTER-AGENCY TASK FORCE ON INFANT FEEDING AND HIV-INFECTED MOTHERS

• When replacement feeding is acceptable, feasible, affordable, sustainable, and safe, avoidance of all breast-feeding by HIV-infected mothers is recommended.

• Otherwise, exclusive breast-feeding is recommended during the first months of life.

• To minimize HIV transmission risk, breast-feeding should be discontinued as soon as feasible, taking into account local circumstances, the individual woman's situation, and the risks of replacement feeding (including infections other than HIV and malnutrition).

• When HIV-infected mothers choose not to breast-feed from birth or stop breast-feeding later, they should be provided with specific guidance and support for at least the first two years of the child's life to ensure adequate replacement feeding. Programs should strive to improve conditions that will make replacement feeding safer for HIV-infected mothers and families.

• HIV-infected mothers who breast-feed should be provided with specific guidance and support when they cease breast-feeding to avoid harmful nutritional and psychological consequences and to maintain breast health.

—UNFPA/UNICEF/WHO/UNAIDS, Inter-Agency Task Team on Mother-to-Child Transmission of HIV, January 15, 2001, *www.unaids.org.*

UNICEF/WHO BABY-FRIENDLY HOSPITAL INITIATIVE: TEN STEPS TO SUCCESSFUL BREAST-FEEDING

To become a baby-friendly hospital, every facility providing maternity services and care for newborn infants should:

1. Have a written breast-feeding policy that is routinely communicated to all health care staff.

2. Train all health care staff in skills necessary to implement this policy.

3. Inform all pregnant women about the benefits and management of breast-feeding.

4. Help mothers initiate breast-feeding within half an hour of birth.

5. Show mothers how to breast-feed, and how to maintain lactation even if they should be separated from their infants.

6. Give newborn infants no food or drink other than breast milk, unless medically indicated.

7. Practice rooming-in—allow mothers and infants to remain together twenty-four-hours a day.

8. Encourage breast-feeding on demand.

9. Give no artificial teats or pacifiers (dummies or soothers) to breast-feeding infants.

10. Foster the establishment of breast-feeding support groups and refer mothers to them on discharge from the hospital or clinic.

to receive subsidized or free formula for six months. But where HIV prevalence is high it will not be possible to supply commercial infant formula for all babies who need it. Care must be taken to ensure that breast-feeding in general is not undermined by the availability of free or subsidized infant formula.

It is possible to make homemade formulas from animal milks, such as cow, buffalo, or goat milk. Unmodified animal milk has too great a proportion of protein and can damage the baby's kidneys and irritate the intestine. It is necessary to dilute the milk with water and to add sugar for energy.

RECIPE FOR COW'S MILK FORMULA FOR A BABY FROM BIRTH TO SIX MONTHS

To make 150 mls of formula:

100 mls of cow's milk
50 mls of water
10 grams (2 teaspoons) of sugar

Boil the mixture.
Such formulas lack micronutrients.

—WHO, UNICEF, UNAIDS, *HIV and Infant Feeding: A Guide for Health Care Managers and Supervisors.* May 1998. WHO/FRH/NT/CD/98.2

HIV is killed easily by heat — the virus dies above 56° C. A woman could express her breast milk, boil it and feed by cup to her baby. Although some of the anti-infective properties are reduced, many important components are unaffected, and heated breast milk is nutritionally superior to other milks. In practice it may be difficult for a woman to express her milk for months without the stimulation of the baby sucking at the breast. However, this is an inexpensive and nutritionally appropriate option, and women may want to try it. They will need support and advice about alternatives in case they are unable to maintain their supply of breast milk. They will also need practical advice about boiling milk (and about other cooking) in a small pan with a lid to avoid small amounts rapidly boiling away.

Whatever replacement is used, it is important that the mother or carer is taught how to use a cup to feed the baby. A cup is simple to clean thoroughly and does not need to be sterilized. Bacteria grow easily in bottles and rubber nipples, which are difficult to clean and need to be boiled before use. Even a newborn baby can cup feed, and cup feeding ensures that the mother or caregiver holds the baby during feeding.

It is possible that a female relative could breast-feed a baby who has an infected mother. In many cultures even post-menopausal grandmothers have relactated in order to feed a baby. (In some countries this must be the paternal grandmother; in others, it is the mother's mother who should feed the baby.) Such traditional solutions can be encouraged. It is important to be sure that "wet-nurses" are not infected with HIV, and they should be counseled about the possibility that if the baby is infected with HIV there is a small risk that it may be transmitted to the wet-nurse.

Supporting the mothers

In many countries, especially in rural areas, breast-feeding is highly valued and is regarded as an important part of mothering by the whole community. Women may find it very difficult not to breast-feed. Girls grow up expecting and looking forward to breast-feeding, a source of pleasure for the mother as well as the baby. A woman who does not breast-feed may meet with social disapproval. She needs to be prepared for this and given support. She may also feel that she is not a good mother and take time to come to terms with choosing not to breast-feed, especially if the decision has been made by a health professional or by her husband or his mother. It will be helpful to emphasize that she is a good mother because she has weighed the risks and made a difficult choice in the best interests of her child. Remind her that there are many things that mothers do for their children; feeding is only one of them. Women who do not breast-feed need to be counseled to expect a rapid return of menses and fertility. Women may also be stigmatized if they are assumed to

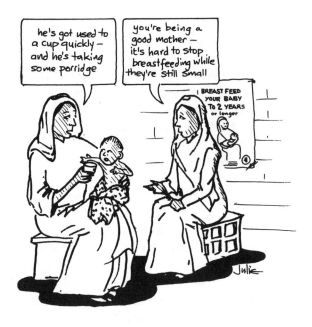

have HIV because they do not breast-feed. Support is also important because in humanitarian settings there are so many mothers without the support of a husband or mother.

Limitations of test-dependent interventions

Access to test-dependent interventions in combination with antiretroviral therapy has reduced the risk of MTCT for positive pregnant women in industrialized countries to less than 4 percent. Several analyses suggest that prenatal VCT and ARVP would be cost-effective in both high- and low-prevalence countries. However, these test-dependent interventions can only avert a limited proportion of HIV infections in children, even when acceptance increases. This is because not all women are able to access prenatal care, and because these interventions miss women who become infected late in pregnancy or in the post-partum period. These women have the highest risk of transmission to their babies because the post-infection peak in viral load inevitably occurs when they are pregnant or lactating.

The potential public health impact of test-dependent interventions is greater in countries with a very low incidence of new infections. ARVP regimens (such as nevirapine) that can be given during labor and post-partum might also improve their potential, although many

women do not deliver in the hospital, and testing for HIV during labor has significant ethical implications. It has been suggested that in high prevalence areas all mothers and babies could be given a single dose of nevirapine without prenatal VCT. This might be a short-term option in humanitarian settings when the prevalence of HIV among pregnant women is known to be high and it is not feasible or safe to introduce VCT during pregnancy.

Rights and ethical considerations

There can be pressure to implement screening for HIV during pregnancy and provide ARVP. This seems like a straightforward and effective intervention. However, there are adverse effects associated with offering HIV testing during pregnancy, and these test-dependent interventions need to be introduced carefully.

Informed consent

When a woman attends prenatal care she is not thinking of having an HIV test, yet may accept when it is offered because she thinks it is expected. In many studies a high proportion of those who agreed to be tested did not return for their results. Women may justifiably fear the consequences of disclosure of their status for themselves and their children, including family conflict, stigma, isolation, fear, secret keeping, expulsion from the family, or violence. This fear may be even greater in camp settings. Sometimes husbands prevent their wives from returning for the results, and the woman then misses out on prenatal and delivery care. In a camp setting it may be more difficult for a pregnant woman to avoid learning the result of an HIV test carried out at the prenatal clinic.

Several countries have introduced group "counseling" before HIV testing in prenatal clinics because of resource constraints and the need to improve coverage. It is important to study the impact of group counseling on informed consent.

There are ethical implications to the introduction in prenatal clinics of rapid tests that provide the results within hours instead of requiring a second visit. Rapid tests may assist those for whom transport is an obstacle but may make it more difficult for women to choose not to receive their result. They should be introduced only where there is confidential and individual (rather than group) pre-test counseling.

In many societies the meaning of "informed consent" may be confusing or problematic. Women, especially young married women, may have little autonomy. They may have no experience of being asked to make important decisions and may feel uncomfortable. Issues of pregnancy, childbirth, and care of babies may also concern the husband, mother-in-law, or extended family. Whether and how they should be included in counseling can best be resolved through consultation with the community.

In humanitarian settings pregnant women may be especially sensitive. The pregnancy may be unwelcome, the result of rape or coerced sex. Women who are pregnant may fear what the future holds for their baby and worry about how they are going to be able to look after a baby in such uncertain times, when they have no home or land. These issues need to be discussed when training prenatal care workers in VCT.

The man's right to information

The majority of HIV-infected pregnant married women have been infected by their husbands, so a positive HIV test result is a "marker" of HIV infection in the husband. When we test a woman we put her in a position where she has a responsibility to inform her husband if she has a positive result. But he has not had the opportunity to receive pre-test counseling and give informed consent to knowing his HIV status. A possible solution to this conflict of rights is to encourage, as a routine, the second prenatal visit to be a "couple visit." This could be promoted in relation to the need to diagnose and treat for infectious diseases generally, rather than a focus on HIV, and to plan for emergency transport for delivery. At this visit the couple could be counseled together and the issue of blame addressed with both present. The visit would also provide an opportunity to give the man information about the risk he presents to his wife and baby if he has unprotected sex outside the marriage while his wife is pregnant or breast-feeding. The woman could be asked

at the first visit whether she is willing to be counseled about testing with her husband.

Care for the mother

The availability of test-dependent interventions leaves us in the awkward position of being able to offer a woman some hope for her child, while leaving her with the knowledge that she has a fatal disease. It is important to include follow-up care and support for the woman and her family when such a program is introduced. This may include counseling, support groups, and providing prophylaxis and treatment for opportunistic infections (see page 179). The reductions in prices of lifelong treatment with combination antiretroviral drugs sharpen ethical concerns about identifying women with HIV during pregnancy. Many countries are starting to offer long-term treatment for HIV infection rather than just prophylaxis to women who test positive for HIV. Noerine Kaleeba, UNAIDS Community Mobilisation Officer, has declared that we should not forget that the most important way to support children is to keep their parents alive: "As long as I am still alive and healthy, I will be able to take care of my children."

Even if it is possible to ensure confidentiality when a woman is tested for HIV, the interventions of ARVP, avoidance of breast-feeding, or caesarean section may reveal her HIV status to others. There is an obligation to allocate resources and effort to the reduction of stigma when plans are made to introduce these interventions.

Women often discover for the first time that they have HIV infection when their baby shows signs and symptoms suggestive of HIV and is tested. It is not ethical to tell her that she should not have any more children. She has a right to information about the risk. But if she is well herself and does not have signs of HIV-related illness, the risk of MTCT is likely to be low. In many societies the desire to have a baby is very strong, and women may have no social role if they are not mothers. Women who have HIV-related signs and symptoms are much more likely to have an infected baby. These women need careful counseling to make sure that they understand the risks and have thought about how the baby would be cared for if they were to die.

STRATEGIES

Resources for prevention and care in relation to PTCT of HIV need to be allocated to both:

- specific primary prevention strategies to prevent new infections during pregnancy and lactation, and

- secondary prevention interventions, including those that do not depend on prenatal VCT, as well as the test-dependent interventions.

These strategies need participation from both men and women in initial assessment of the situation and planning, as well as in implementing and evaluation. Integrate strategies with existing community-based programs, rather than establishing separate structures and processes. Page 157 shows a framework to aid discussion. Key steps for an integrated PTCT response are as follows:

Gather information relevant to the successful implementation of PTCT prevention and care strategies

This should include rapid qualitative studies using key informant interviews and focus group discussions of attitudes, knowledge, and practice in relation to:

- VCT during pregnancy (meaning of "informed choice," involvement of husband and family, confidentiality);

- consequences of a woman disclosing a positive HIV test result;

- contraception;

- prenatal care;

- influences on exclusive breast-feeding;

- pre-emergency infant feeding knowledge and practice;

- feasible alternatives to breast-feeding;

- current weaning food practices; and

- care of sick babies and orphans.

If possible, an estimate of the number of pregnant women in the beneficiary population is useful for planning.

Prevent new infections during pregnancy, post-partum, lactation

- Promote the idea of planning for pregnancy.

- Improve access to VCT (outside pregnancy) for couples.

- Introduce a routine evening "couple" prenatal visit.

- Promote condoms.

- Strengthen management of STIs.

- Train midwives in active management of the third stage of labor to reduce the need for transfusions and to implement strict transfusion criteria.

- Train health care workers to advise fathers after delivery that unprotected sex with others carries a high risk of infection of HIV to their baby; provide condoms.

- Develop IEC campaign and materials to support these activities, especially addressing men.

- Train health care workers to advise discordant couples *if they are eager to conceive* how to minimize the risk of transmission to woman and baby by teaching women how to recognize the timing of ovulation so they need to have unprotected intercourse only once each month.

Strengthen reproductive health services for secondary prevention interventions (not dependent on HIV testing)

- Prevent unwanted pregnancies.

- Encourage planning of pregnancies.

- Train health workers to counsel women with any chronic illness to avoid pregnancy until well for six months.

- Promote quality prenatal care with treatment of STIs and with other infections and nutrition advice.

INTEGRATING PTCT STRATEGIES WITH MATERNAL AND REPRODUCTIVE HEALTH WORK

IRC supports health centers near Bukavu in the Democratic Republic of the Congo. One of these is the well-managed Mugeri health center, which has in-patient beds, caring and motivated staff, clean rooms, protocols, and posters on the walls, and is popular with patients. The nurse in charge, Mr. Nyankwega, said he regretted that they could do nothing to prevent mother-to-child transmission (MTCT) of HIV. In fact he and his staff are doing a great deal to prevent MTCT: they are providing good prenatal care and involving the husbands; they are distributing condoms and other ways of contraception; they are treating sexually transmitted infections (STIs); they rupture membranes and perform episiotomies only when strictly necessary; and they keep new mothers for five days so they have a chance to rest and establish exclusive breast-feeding.

A father was sitting in a postnatal room proudly holding his new baby. This would be a good time to explain to men that unprotected sex would put them at risk of HIV, and they would then have a very high risk of infecting their wife and baby. He agreed that new fathers had a right to the information and would be receptive because they feel responsible and loving at this time. They could introduce a routine evening "couple visit" as the second prenatal visit, at which any infections could be diagnosed and treated, couples could be counseled and tested together, men could be informed of the risks they pose to their baby if they have unsafe sex during or after the pregnancy, and emergency transport plans for labor could be discussed. The center's staff could also be trained to advise any women who had a chronic illness to avoid pregnancy until they had been well for six months, since the risk that HIV will pass to the baby is high when an infected pregnant woman is ill.

These measures to reduce the number of HIV-infected babies in this population are feasible. They address the factors that we know increase the risk of transmission; they do not depend on identification of women who are infected with HIV; and they improve the health of men and women generally.

- Train midwives and traditional birth attendants to reduce unnecessary obstetric interventions.

- Establish strict criteria for transfusion.

- Promote exclusive breast-feeding.

- Train health care workers in breast-feeding to minimize breast problems.

Prepare for the introduction of test-dependent interventions

Test-dependent interventions (prenatal VCT, ARVP, HIV, and infant feeding counseling and, when feasible, elective caesarean section) should be introduced in humanitarian settings only if the following are in place:

- well-functioning maternal and child health services;

- accessible and acceptable VCT services;

- quality and confidential testing facilities;

- a sustainable supply of antiretroviral drugs;

- community acceptance of those infected and affected by HIV; and

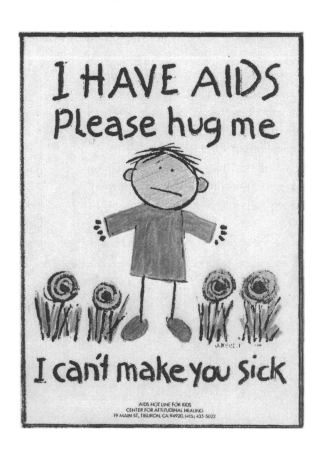

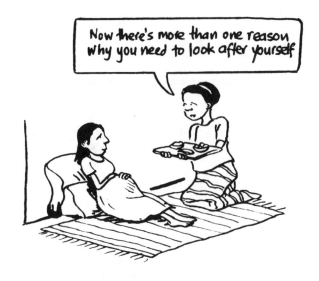

- the resources for low-cost follow-up care and support of infected mothers, babies, and their families. Although long-term antiretroviral therapy may not yet be affordable, it is important to ensure access to prevention and treatment of opportunistic infections.

It will also be necessary to train health care workers and midwives in VCT and counseling for HIV and infant feeding (see the counseling checklist on page 152).

If refugees and IDPs come from a setting with a high prevalence of HIV and where testing was available there may be pregnant women who already know that they are HIV-positive. In these situations it is helpful to have a supply of antiretroviral drugs available for prophylaxis, even though it may not be possible to implement a full ARVP program.

Where termination of pregnancy is legal and feasible, health workers may need to be trained in discussing this option with HIV-positive women. Health workers may feel that HIV-positive women should be encouraged to terminate their pregnancy because (1) the baby may become infected with HIV, and (2) the baby will one day be an orphan. It is important to point out to these workers that when the mother is well the risk to the baby may be quite small and that their concern that the child may be orphaned is not an ethical reason to encourage a woman to terminate a wanted pregnancy.

Develop an IEC community campaign

Men's role in protection of their family and their desire for healthy children suggests that appeals to their sense of responsibility may be a powerful trigger to behavior change. An IEC campaign needs to disseminate the following messages:

- Plan for pregnancy; first seek VCT, treat any infections, improve nutrition.

- Prevent unwanted pregnancies; use contraception.

- Seek information about PTCT of HIV.

- Support mothers caring for sick babies; they need sympathy, not blame, from family and community.

- Give love and attention to children with HIV; they do not spread the virus to others.

- Take advantage of prenatal care to help you have a healthy pregnancy and avoid complications.

- Attend the second prenatal visit together as a couple.

- Give the best food to the woman when she is pregnant, and make sure that she does not work too hard.

- Use condoms (appeal to men's sense of responsibility and desire to protect the family).

- Avoid unprotected sex during or after the pregnancy; it can harm the baby.

- Consider attending VCT as a couple.

- Breast-feed exclusively for six months; this is best for all babies,

- Postpone pregnancy if you are ill; wait until well for six months before becoming pregnant.

Awareness that HIV also affects babies may act as a stimulus for young people to protect themselves and encourage communities to mobilize to care for orphans and sick children.

In this rapidly changing field it is important to keep up to date. The Inter-Agency Task Force publishes frequent updates available on the UNAIDS website (*www.unaids.org*).

CHECKLIST FOR COUNSELING ON HIV
AND INFANT FEEDING

[It is best if counseling for HIV and infant feeding does not take place at the same time as post-test counseling when the result has been positive. It will be difficult for the woman to take in information about the different risks and make a decision when she has just heard that she is HIV-positive. Refer to the checklist for post-test counseling on page 81. Tell her that there are actions that she can take to lessen the risk to the baby and arrange a suitable time to discuss them with her.]

- Introduce yourself.

- Explain that the interview is completely confidential.

- Explain that the purpose of the interview is to provide information about HIV and infant feeding and to help the woman to reach a decision about the safest way for her to feed her baby.

- Ask whether she knows her HIV status. She may have had a test and so knows her status. If she has not had a test ask her how likely she thinks it is that she may be infected. She may have no reason to think that she is infected. On the other hand she may have good reason to believe that she is infected, for example, her husband may have AIDS, she may have HIV-related symptoms and signs, or her previous child may have died. In areas of high prevalence this situation is likely to be common. What the woman thinks about her likely risk of infection will influence her decisions about how to feed her baby. This discussion may lead her to think again about having an HIV test, and it may be helpful to explore her reasons for not wanting to be tested. In particular, ask her whether it might be possible for her husband to come for counseling so that they could be tested together.

- Check her understanding about HIV infection and mother-to-child transmission.

- Correct any false beliefs and provide information about HIV and infant feeding.

- Make a set of cards to assist in counseling. Each card has one of the following points (written in the local language) and illustrated with an appropriate picture. The counselor then explains each card in turn to the woman and asks questions to find out about the woman's own situation. Key points:

  - Breast-feeding is very important to child health, particularly for the first six months. It provides all the nutrients the baby needs and protects against infections, especially diarrhea. Breast-feeding helps mothers and babies to feel close and warm.

  - Breast-feeding protects a woman from becoming pregnant again quickly. Women who do not breast-feed have monthly periods again soon after the birth.

  - Breast-feeding is the most convenient and cheapest way to feed a baby. It is difficult to provide an alternative to breast-feeding if you have to travel with a baby.

CHECKLIST FOR COUNSELING ON HIV
AND INFANT FEEDING (CONTINUED)

- Breast-feeding carries a risk of transmission of HIV. About one-third of babies who have an HIV-positive mother will become infected with HIV. The virus is most likely to pass to the baby during labor or in the first few weeks of breast-feeding, although a small proportion become infected earlier in the pregnancy. If 100 HIV-infected pregnant women have a baby, we expect that about 7 of the babies will become infected in the womb, about 15 of them at the time of delivery, and about 13 of them through breast-feeding (show picture). But we cannot tell at birth which babies are already infected with HIV. We also cannot say what the risk is for one particular woman. If a woman has no HIV-related symptoms and her HIV infection is not recent, she may have a lower risk than a woman who is ill or recently infected with HIV.

- The risk of transmission through breast-feeding is greatest in the early weeks, but remains throughout the duration of breast-feeding—even into the second year of life.

- Exclusive breast-feeding carries a lower risk than mixed feeding and may provide some protection against transmission of HIV that occurs at the time of delivery. Exclusive breast-feeding means that the baby receives nothing but breast milk.

- Most babies born to HIV-infected mothers who are breast fed do not become infected with HIV and may benefit from antibodies in the breast milk.

- The risk is greater if the mother has signs and symptoms of HIV infection, especially if she is already ill with AIDS. The risk is lower if the mother is well.

- The risk is higher if there are any breast problems such as cracked nipples, engorgement, mastitis, or breast abscess, or if the baby has thrush in the mouth.

• If the woman is HIV negative or does not know her HIV status, recommend that she breast-feed exclusively for six months and then continue to breast-feed while introducing appropriate weaning foods. If she has not been tested, discuss with her the possibility of an HIV test and discuss whether she might like to ask her husband to come for counseling and testing.

• If the woman knows that she is HIV positive, recommend that she avoid breast-feeding if it is possible for her to give an adequate replacement, or breast-feed exclusively for four to six months and then stop breast-feeding if safe weaning foods are available. Point out to the woman that she does not need to decide everything about how she will feed the baby at this stage. Before the birth she needs to decide whether she will breast-feed at all. After the baby is born, it will be both difficult and unwise to reverse a decision not to breast-feed at all. If she decides to breast-feed she should breast-feed exclusively. She may later decide to stop breast-feeding and give a replacement, for example, if her circumstances become more stable and she is confident that she will have an adequate alternative. On the other hand she may have planned to stop breast-feeding at six months—but if the baby is showing signs of HIV infection she may decide the best course of action is to continue to breast-feed. Then her baby can have the benefits of breast milk for as long as possible to minimize the recurrent infections and to provide comfort when the baby is ill.

CHECKLIST FOR COUNSELING ON HIV
AND INFANT FEEDING (CONTINUED)

- Help her to weigh up the risks relevant to her own situation. The idea of weighing up risks can be difficult for a woman to understand. Her choice is not a simple one of deciding whether the risk of death for her baby is greater if she breast-feeds than if she does not. Her decision will be influenced by many factors. Some she may tell you; some she may keep private. This is why it is important that the woman makes the decision and not the counselor. You can ask her the following questions to help her to decide.

    – What will be the most difficult problems if you decide not to breast-feed?

       • Do you have an affordable and accessible supply of cow's milk and sugar or of infant formula that will continue to be available for at least six months?

       • Will you be able to boil water or milk?

       • Will you be able to prepare feeds in a clean way in your present circumstances?

       • Will you have time to feed the baby?

       • Is there anyone who will be able to help you to feed the baby?

       • What do you think your family, friends, and neighbors will say if you don't breast-feed?

       • How will you feel yourself if you don't breast-feed?

       • What will you do if you have to travel with your baby and the baby is not breast-feeding?

       • What will you do about feeding the baby during the night?

       • What will you do if your husband or other children are hungry and ask for the baby's milk?

    – What will make it difficult to exclusively breast-feed (nothing but breast milk, including no water)?

       • Is there a belief that colostrum is harmful?

       • Are newborn babies routinely given water?

       • Is there a belief that it is important to give herbs or medicines or any other fluid before the breast milk "comes in"?

       • Who makes the decision about when to give the baby foods in addition to breast milk?

       • Are there times when you have to leave the baby and some other milk or foods are usually given?

- Give advice about storing, preparing, and feeding weaning foods, since babies who are not breast-feeding have a higher risk of diarrheal disease.

- Whatever the woman decides, reassure her that she has thought carefully about the best decision for her baby. Check her understanding. Tell her that she can return if she has any questions or difficulties. If she is literate give her appropriate written information.

- Ask about family circumstances and identify what support she has from family and friends

- If the woman decides not to breast-feed, arrange a follow-up appointment before the birth so that you can show her how to prepare a feed, and she can practice this.

HIV INFECTION OF BABIES

One hundred pregnant HIV positive women

On average thirty-five babies will be infected with HIV

Seven become infected during the pregnancy

Fifteen become infected at the time of delivery

Thirteen become infected through breastfeeding – most in the early weeks

SUGGESTED INDICATORS

Indicator	*Method of measurement*
PTCT interventions informed by an understanding of relevant attitudes, knowledge, and practices	Qualitative study report
Proportion of pregnant women attending for prenatal care	Survey
Proportion of husbands attending at least one prenatal clinic visit	Survey/review of clinic attendance records
Proportion of pregnant women using condoms	Survey
Midwives trained and competent in active management of third stage of labor and criteria for transfusion	Review of training reports/ supervision checklists
Proportion of births in clinic/hospital where the father has been counseled about risks of unprotected sex	Review of clinic/hospital records
IEC materials developed and disseminated	Review of materials and records
Decrease in artificial rupture of membranes, and transfusions at delivery	Review of hospital/clinic records
Proportion of mothers of babies over four months who exclusively breast-fed for at least four months	Survey
Increase in community knowledge about PTCT	Survey results compared to baseline/focus group discussion findings
Number of health care workers trained in HIV and infant feeding counseling	Review of training records
HIV and infant feeding counseling checklist developed and available	Observation

CONCEPTUALIZING PREVENTION OF PARENT-TO-CHILD TRANSMISSION OF HIV

PRIMARY PREVENTION (prevent infection of women and men)		SECONDARY PREVENTION (prevent virus passing from infected women to infants)	
Nonspecific interventions	**Specific interventions**	**Non-test-dependent interventions**	**Specific test-dependent interventions**
(prevent transmission between men and women)	*(prevent new infections during pregnancy, delivery, and lactation)*	*(do not depend on testing during pregnancy)*	*(depend on knowledge of women's HIV status)*
For example:	• Introduce as routine an evening "couple" visit as the second prenatal visit, for discussion of screening for and prevention of infections (TB, STIs, HIV), and preparing for labor.	• Prevent unwanted pregnancies:	Provide VCT for pregnant women. For those HIV positive offer:
• Reduce stigma and discrimination.		– Increase access to VCT and contraception	• Antiretroviral prophylaxis
• Increase community capacity for behavior change (e.g., Stepping Stones approach).	• Counsel fathers after delivery, or at ceremonies to celebrate the birth, that unprotected sex with others carries a high risk of infection of HIV to their baby; provide condoms.	– Community education	• HIV and infant feeding counseling to assist women to make a choice between exclusive breast-feeding or exclusive replacement feeding based on individual risk assessment, and follow-up support
• Provide access to quality VCT for men, women, and couples.	• Train midwives in active management of the third stage of labor to reduce need for transfusions and implement strict transfusion criteria.	• Encourage women with any chronic illness to avoid pregnancy until well for six months	
• Develop peer education.	• Community education about PTCT, especially addressing men.	• Improve health of pregnant and lactating women:	
• Promote and distribute female and male condoms.	• Help discordant couples if they are eager to conceive to minimize the risk of transmission to woman and baby; improve access to VCT for both men and women; counsel couples about timing of ovulation so they need have unprotected intercourse only once each month; diagnose and treat STIs.	– Promote quality ANC; treat STIs and other infections; nutrition advice	• Elective caesarean section (if appropriate)
• Improve management of STIs.		– Community education	
• Behavior change communication with youth.		• Reduce risk of transmission at delivery:	• Counseling re termination of pregnancy (if appropriate, where legal)
• Address the problem of sexual abuse of children.	• Counsel women/couples when a woman tests negative for HIV during pregnancy.	– Train midwives to reduce unnecessary artificial rupture of membranes and episiotomies	• Post-partum counseling re contraception choices
		• Reduce risk of transmission through breast-feeding:	
		– Promote exclusive breast-feeding	
		– Train health care workers in breast-feeding to minimize breast problems; treat infant oral thrush	

ADDITIONAL RESOURCES

Emergency Nutrition Network. *Infant Feeding in Emergencies: Policy, Strategy, and Practice.* For policy makers. Report of the Ad Hoc Group on Infant Feeding in Emergencies, May 1999. Also: *Infant Feeding in Emergencies: Module 1.* For emergency relief staff. March 2001. *www.tcd.ie.*

Holmes, W., and T. Kwarteng. "Parent to Child Transmission of HIV: Policy Considerations in the Asia-Pacific Region," *Journal of Clinical Virology* 22 (2001): 315–24.

UN Inter-Agency Task Team on Mother-to-Child Transmission of HIV. "New Data on the Prevention of Mother-to-Child Transmission of HIV and Their Policy Implications: Conclusions and Recommendations." Geneva, October 11–13, 2000; published January 15, 2001. Available at *www.unaids.org.*

WHO, UNICEF, UNAIDS. *HIV and Infant Feeding: A Guide for Health Care Managers and Supervisors.* May 1998. Available from Programme of Nutrition, WHO, Geneva, Switzerland, at the UNAIDS website: *www.unaids.org* (WHO/FRH/NT/CD/98.2).

WHO. *Infant Feeding in Emergencies.* For mothers. Prepared for the Programme for Nutrition Policy, Infant Feeding and Food Security Lifestyles and Health Unit, World Health Organization Regional Office for Europe, Copenhagen. World Health Organization, Regional Office for Europe EU/ICP/LVNG 01 02 08. Revised September 1997. Available at *www.who.dk.*

12

Prevention of Transmission through Blood Transfusion

Blood transfusions can save lives, but in areas where HIV is prevalent and the rate of new infections is high, they may result in transmission of HIV or other blood-borne infections. Armed conflict often gives rise to the need for blood transfusions. In the post-emergency phase childbirth, trauma, and severe anemia due to malaria may necessitate transfusion.

RATIONALE

Transmission through transfusion of blood or blood products is preventable. Since 1985 it has been possible to test donated blood for HIV antibodies. Routine testing of all blood for transfusion greatly reduces the chances of transmitting HIV but a small risk remains. This is because donors can give blood after infection, but before they develop antibodies and before the test has become positive — the "window period." The risk is greatest in areas where many people are becoming infected with HIV.

To reduce the risk of infection through transfusion:

1. Reduce unnecessary use of blood transfusion by introducing and monitoring strict transfusion criteria and training in use of blood substitutes.

2. Reduce the risk that blood donors are infected with HIV through careful selection of donors.

3. Establish routine screening for HIV, syphilis, hepatitis B, and, if funds permit, hepatitis C.

4. Encourage the use of autologous blood transfusions[1] whenever possible.

_____
1. Autologous blood transfusion is the collection and subsequent reinfusion of the patient's own blood or blood components.

In humanitarian settings there should be persons nominated to organize a safe blood supply. They will need to consult with the local health authorities, for example, the district or provincial medical officer, and, if there is one, the local blood transfusion service officer. Is there a National Blood Transfusion Service blood policy and plan? How well does the Blood Transfusion Service function locally? Are blood donors paid or volunteers? Is there a system for selecting donors and excluding those who may be at risk of HIV infection? What infections, if any, is the blood screened for? Are there criteria for transfusion? Is there a campaign to recruit volunteer blood donors? The local service may need upgrading; in rural or remote settings a new system may need to be established. Donated blood can be stored for up to thirty-five days at a constant temperature between 2°C and 8°C. Often it is not possible to set up a blood bank in humanitarian settings, but procedures for safe transfusion and training of health staff are essential. Efforts should be made to ensure that the local host population also has access to a safe blood supply.

STRATEGIES

Reduce unnecessary use of blood transfusion by introducing and monitoring strict transfusion criteria

Even when blood is screened it is important to transfuse blood only when absolutely necessary. Fresh whole blood or red blood cells are usually transfused because of blood loss, for example, during surgery, trauma, childbirth, gastrointestinal bleeding, or ruptured ectopic pregnancy, or for severe anemia, most commonly due to malaria. Anemia due to malaria is the most common reason for children to receive a transfusion in sub-Saharan Africa. Studies show that many transfusions were not needed. Several studies have found that strict criteria for blood transfusion can greatly reduce the number of transfusions without any increase in mortality or morbidity.[2] Many patients can tolerate low levels of hemoglobin without transfusion. Normal saline or colloid solutions instead of blood can often be infused for acute blood loss to maintain blood pressure until the bleeding can be stopped.[3] Effective treatment and control of malaria, and training midwives in active management of the third stage of labor are also important ways to reduce the need for transfusions.

If these criteria are followed, transfusions could be reduced by over 50 percent without increasing mortality. Doctors in Kinshasa found that by following strict criteria they reduced transfusions by 75 percent without any increase in deaths.[4]

Training health professionals to minimize transfusions is essential; monitoring is also needed. The reason for a transfusion should always be documented. Doctors often believe what they were originally taught and may resist adopting new criteria. In some East European countries some children became infected with HIV because of the common practice of giving "micro" transfusions to children to strengthen them.

Reduce the risk that blood donors are infected with HIV through careful selection of donors

In some countries volunteers or family members donate most blood for transfusion. In others people are paid to donate their blood. These professional blood donors may be at higher risk

for HIV. For example, injecting drug users may sell their blood to get money for drugs. Paid donors may donate blood frequently, which is a risk to their health.

A system of registered voluntary donors is the safest but is likely to be difficult to achieve if the population has not experienced voluntary donation in their own country. When family members donate blood, there can be problems with confidentiality in relation to testing — and family members may be less likely than anonymous volunteers to provide information about possible exposures to HIV. Nevertheless they may be the only option. Where there is no blood banking, donors may need to be selected case by case.

Community education about the value and responsibility of blood donation can encourage those who may be at risk of HIV or other blood-borne viruses to exclude themselves from donation. This education should include the message that blood donation should not be used as a way to find out your HIV status.

A questionnaire needs to be developed for potential donors. Experience suggests that it is helpful if a trained health care worker can go through the interview with each potential donor. The questionnaire should include questions about:

- sexual activities,

- ear and skin piercing,

- tattoos or traditional skin incisions,

- injecting drug use and sharing of injecting equipment,

- recent illnesses, including sexually transmitted infections,

- family history of illness,

- previous transfusions of blood or a blood product,

- previous blood donations (including if paid),

- general health and nutrition.

This information must be kept strictly confidential and the potential donor must be told this. Individuals should be asked not to give blood if they may have been at risk of HIV.

2. NHMRC, "Clinical Practice Guidelines on the Appropriate Use of Red Blood Cells," December 12, 2000, National Health and Medical Research Council and the Australasian Society of Blood Transfusion, *www.health.gov.au/nhmrc*.

3. WHO, *Global Blood Safety Initiative: Use of Plasma Substitutes and Plasma in Developing Countries* (Geneva: WHO, 1989), WHO/GPA/INF/89.17.

4. F. Davachi et al., "Effects of an Educational Campaign to Reduce Blood Transfusions in Children in Kinshasa, Zaire." Fifth International Conference on AIDS, Montreal, 1989.

CRITERIA FOR BLOOD TRANSFUSIONS

CRITERIA FOR TRANSFUSION BECAUSE OF BLOOD LOSS

In previously healthy patients with acute blood loss of less than 1000 mls:

- Control the bleeding.
- Give a non-blood plasma volume expander such as dextran 70 or polygeline. If not available infuse normal saline (0.9 percent) or Ringer's Lactate solution.

Restoring volume is more important than replacing oxygen-carrying capacity so a transfusion is not necessary unless active bleeding continues with loss in excess of 1000 mls and signs of shock (low blood pressure and rapid pulse rate). Loss of over 40 percent of blood volume is life-threatening and requires transfusion of blood, if available.

CRITERIA FOR TRANSFUSION BECAUSE OF ANEMIA

- Hemoglobin is less than 7 g/dl with symptoms: edema, dizziness, shortness of breath, tiredness, rapid heart rate.
- Hemoglobin is less than 6 g/dl, even without symptoms.
- Angina pectoris with hemoglobin less than 10 g/dl.
- Before an operation: hemoglobin is less than 7 g/dl and the surgical blood loss is likely to be greater than 500 mls.

  Find and treat the cause of the anemia. Give iron and folate.

For children under twelve years with severe anemia due to malaria, the benefit from transfusion depends on the timing of the transfusion, hemoglobin concentration, and clinical status. Transfusions have been found to be beneficial only if given within the first two days of admission. In those with severe anemia, transfusion may be harmful because of volume overload in those who are already hemodynamically compromised.

Transfusion is indicated if:

- Hb < 5.0 g/dl and there are symptoms and signs of congestive heart failure (breathlessness, rapid pulse, edema).
- Hb < 3.0 g/dl without symptoms and signs.

—WHO, *The Clinical Use of Blood Handbook* (Geneva: WHO, 2001).

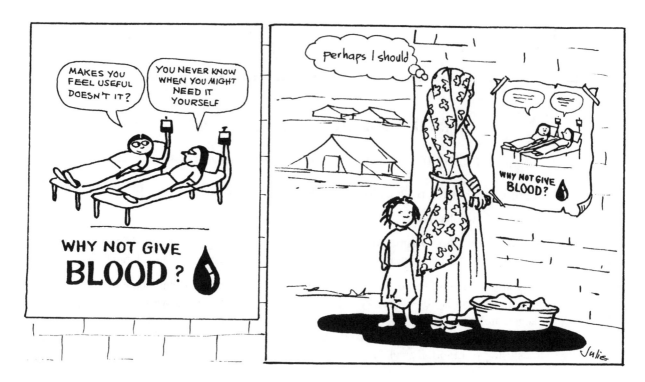

When feasible it is important to develop a system for registering donors and to make efforts to motivate and retain low-risk donors.

Establish routine screening of blood for transfusion

All blood for transfusion must always be screened for HIV, syphilis, hepatitis B, and, if funds permit, hepatitis C. Rhesus testing and simple ABO compatibility testing before transfusion should also be carried out.

Linked or unlinked screening?

In humanitarian settings confidentiality assumes even greater significance than in stable settings. Unless confidential pre- and post-test counseling by well-trained counselors and confirmatory tests are available, then screening of blood for transfusion should be anonymous and unlinked, that is, the test specimen and the donated blood are labeled with a common identity code, but not with the donor's name, and the donor does not receive the result.

However, if it is feasible to provide counseling and confirmatory testing, then potential donors should receive information explaining the procedure for blood donation, including the need for screening for HIV. At the same time

that the trained health workers conduct the risk history assessment described above, they can:

- check the donor's understanding of how HIV spreads,
- correct any misconceptions,
- describe how to protect against the spread of HIV,
- explain about the length of time before they receive the result, the window period, and confidentiality, and
- obtain informed consent.

Tests

The ELISA test is most commonly used for screening blood for transfusion (see page 90 for a discussion of HIV antibody tests). Dual infection with HIV-1 and HIV-2 may occur, so test kits that can detect both are necessary for screening of blood.

Reduction of the costs of screening

Several strategies can help to reduce the cost of HIV antibody testing. The strategy used for screening blood for transfusion depends on whether or not the donors will be informed of the results.

If the screening is anonymous and unlinked, that is, the donors will not be told the results, then only one test is needed. All serum is tested with one ELISA or simple/rapid assay. Serum that is reactive (gives a positive result) is considered HIV antibody positive, and the blood is destroyed. Serum that is nonreactive is considered HIV antibody negative, and the blood can be transfused.

It is possible to pool several specimens of sera and test them together. If the pooled samples test positive each sample is then tested to find out which was positive. To maintain a high sensitivity the recommended pool size is five samples.

Some countries have developed their own local production facilities for low-cost HIV antibody tests to reduce transport costs and the need for foreign exchange. WHO and UNAIDS help national governments and agencies to obtain high-quality kits at low cost through international tendering for bulk purchases. The list of evaluated test kits and program criteria are available from the blood safety unit at WHO.[5]

If the donors will be told their result then it is necessary to confirm an initial positive result with another different test to be sure that the first result was not a false positive. If the initial test result was negative, this can be reported to the donor, who should receive post-test counseling. If both test results are positive the individuals can be told they are infected with HIV and receive post-test counseling (see page 81).

However, if the first test result is positive and the second test result is negative, further testing is necessary before the donor can be given a result. Of course any donated blood should not be transfused and should be destroyed, whatever the results of confirmatory tests.

Studies have shown that combinations of ELISA and simple/rapid assays for confirmation can provide results as or more reliable than using the more expensive Western Blot confirmatory test. UNAIDS and WHO recommend three testing strategies according to

test objective and prevalence of infection in the population, to maximize accuracy while minimizing cost (see appendix B, page 199).[6]

Encourage the use of autologous blood transfusions whenever possible[7]

Autologous blood transfusion is the collection and subsequent reinfusion of the patient's own blood or blood components. Such transfusions avoid the problem of allergic reactions to blood transfusions, and minimize the use of limited supplies of donated blood.

Before elective operations in which substantial blood loss may occur it is possible to take and store the patient's own blood for use at the time of the operation if adequate blood storage facilities are available. It is safe to take 500 mls at three weeks, two weeks, and one week before surgery in citrate-phosphate-dextrose-adenine to prevent clotting. (Take only 400 mls if the adult weighs less than 50 kgs.) Patients should have a hemoglobin level greater than 10 g/dl (or hematocrit > 30 percent) before their blood is taken. Give oral iron. Label carefully and store the blood in a section of the refrigerator separate from donated blood.

Blood can be removed from a patient immediately prior to surgery with simultaneous replacement by infusion of normal saline solution (3 mls for each ml of blood collected) to maintain the circulating volume. This technique is especially useful where there are no facilities for storage of blood. It does not require specialized equipment other than standard blood bags and transfusion sets. During surgery the patient will lose fewer red blood cells for a given blood loss. The collected blood can be reinfused, after bleeding ceases, which replenishes the patient's hemoglobin, clotting factors, and platelets. The total volume of blood collected should not exceed 40 percent of the patient's estimated blood volume. The blood should be collected into standard plastic blood packs containing citrate-phosphate-dextrose, numbered, and labeled, and should remain with the patient

5. WHO, "Comparative Evaluation of the Operational Characteristics of Commercially Available Assays to Detect Antibodies to HIV-1 and/or HIV-2 in Human Sera," 1991–99, *www.who.int.*

6. *Weekly Epidemiological Record* 21 (March 1997) 72(12), *www.who.int.*

7. WHO/GPA, WHO Health Laboratory Technology and Blood Safety Unit, "Autologous Blood Transfusion in Developing Countries," WHO/GPA/INF/91.1, December 1990; WHO website: Blood Safety and Clinical Technology, *www.who.int/bct/.*

until reinfused. Amounts should be carefully documented, and blood pressure and pulse should be monitored during the procedure. A blood administration set with a standard filter should be used.

Intraoperative blood salvage is the collection of shed blood from a wound or body cavity during surgery and its subsequent reinfusion into the same patient. This can be useful during surgery for ruptured ectopic pregnancy, ruptured spleen, some orthopedic procedures, and traumatic penetrating injuries. Blood should not be salvaged if there has been perforation of the intestine. During the operation the surgeon collects blood from the body cavity using a ladle or small bowl and transfers it into a larger bowl or kidney dish containing acid-citrate-dextrose anticoagulant. Tilting the head of the patient down can assist this process. The blood is then filtered into a sterile bottle through four to six layers of sterile gauze placed in a funnel. The bottle is sealed with the stopper and reinfused through a blood infusion set with a standard filter. Adverse effects are rare.

ADDITIONAL RESOURCES

HIV Testing: A Practical Approach. London: Healthlink Worldwide, 1999.

UNAIDS. "Blood Safety and HIV UNAIDS Technical Update October 1997," *http://unaids.org/publications/ documents/health/index.html#blood*.

Wake, D. J., and W. A. Cutting. "Blood Transfusion in Developing Countries: Problems, Priorities and Practicalities," *Tropical Doctor* 28 (January 1998): 4–8.

SUGGESTED INDICATORS

Indicator	*Method of measurement*
Blood safety officer designated	Document review
Blood safety system established and procedures documented	Document review Observation with checklist
Donor education campaign conducted	Community FGDs Donor interviews
Register of volunteer donors established or case-by-case selection of donors documented	Document review
Self-exclusion questionnaire developed	Review of questionnaire
Proportion of health workers trained to interview, counsel, and exclude donors at risk of HIV	Review of training reports Observation with performance checklists
All blood for transfusion screened for HIV antibodies, syphilis, and other relevant infections	Review of training reports
Procedures to ensure confidentiality established and monitored — or — unlinked anonymous testing in place	Observation with performance checklists
HIV test kits stored securely	Observation checklist Interviews with staff
Transfusion criteria documented and disseminated to relevant health personnel	Observation
Proportion of relevant health professionals trained in use of strict transfusion criteria	Review of training report
System in place to monitor number of transfusions and their indications	Review of documents

13

Prevention of Transmission in Health Care Settings

If proper precautions are not taken, HIV may spread from one patient to another, from a patient to a health care worker, or from a health care worker to a patient.

Fortunately HIV does not spread casually. This means that there is no need for isolation practices or "barrier nursing" of HIV-infected patients, unless they have a contagious opportunistic infection such as infectious diarrhea.

It is natural for health care workers to worry that they may become infected with HIV from their patients. Health staff need clear information about findings from studies of the risk of transmission in health care settings and the factors that increase risk.

RATIONALE

What is the risk of occupational transmission?

The risk of occupational transmission of HIV depends on the prevalence of HIV in the patient population, the chance of becoming infected after a single exposure, and the type and number of exposures.

HIV can be found in blood, semen, vaginal and cervical secretions, urine and feces, wound secretions, saliva, tears, breast milk, and other fluids inside the body. But blood is the only fluid that has been associated with transmission in the health care setting.

Health care workers worry about needle-stick injuries, cuts, getting blood on sores or broken skin, and blood splashes in the eye or mouth. We can reassure them that their risk of infection with HIV through their work is extremely small. Analysis of results from twenty-one studies in developed countries and

Brazil showed a 0.25 percent risk of infection (1 in 400) after a needle-stick injury from an infected patient.[1] The average risk after a mucous membrane exposure (e.g., eye splashes) was only 0.09 percent. When researchers analyzed two hundred incident reports from hospital workers in Thailand who had occupational exposure to HIV-infected blood and body fluids during 1991–97, none of the workers had become infected with HIV.[2] It is also reassuring to note that in places where HIV is common, such as Zaire, studies have found that HIV infection is no more common in health care workers than in the general population.[3]

Although the risk is very small, needle-stick injuries from an HIV-infected person are more likely to lead to HIV infection than splashes or skin contamination. The risk is higher when the needle or cannula has been in the patient's artery or vein, rather than used for an intramuscular injection, when the needle is visibly contaminated with the patient's blood, when the patient is ill with AIDS, and when the injury is deep.[4]

---

1. G. Ippolito et al., "The Risk of Occupational HIV Infection in Health Care Workers," *Archives of Internal Medicine* 153 (1993): 1451–58.

2. P. Phanuphak, K. Pungpapong, and K. Ruxrungtham, "The Risk of Occupational HIV Exposure among Thai Healthcare Workers," *Southeast Asian Journal of Tropical Medicine and Public Health* 30 (1999): 496–503.

3. J. M. Mann et al., "HIV Seroprevalence among Hospital Workers in Kinshasa, Zaire: Lack of Association with Occupational Exposure," *Journal of the American Medical Association* 256 (1986): 3099–3102.

4. G. Ippolito et al., "Occupational Human Immunodeficiency Virus Infection in Health Care Workers: Worldwide Cases through September 1997," *Clinical Infectious Diseases* 28 (1999): 365–83. See also D. M. Cardo et al., "A Case-control Study of HIV Seroconversion in Health Care Workers after Percutaneous Exposure. Centers for Disease Control and Prevention Needlestick Surveillance Group," *New England Journal of Medicine* 337 (1997): 1485–90.

☆ DISCUSSION POINT ☆

How do health care workers behave when they are not well informed about the routes of transmission of HIV and the level of risk of transmission in the health care setting? What effects does this have?

Fear might make health care workers sit at a distance from patients and not touch them. They might arrange for patients to be isolated from others. They might take unnecessary measures such as wearing a mask or gloves during a consultation or fumigating the room afterward. They might insist on testing patients for HIV before surgery, or test for HIV without obtaining informed consent. They might refuse to care for an HIV-infected patient, or to undertake surgery or deliver a baby.

The impact of the behavior of uninformed health care workers can be considerable. Everyone has the same right to nondiscriminatory care and to health care services. People living with HIV are likely to feel hurt and rejected. They may feel angry, or frightened and helpless. If they are refused treatment or surgery their health will be affected. The behavior of the health worker will be observed by others and contribute to fear and stigma associated with people living with HIV in the community. People will be less willing to be tested for HIV if they know that they will be discriminated against and less willing to be open about it if they have been tested already. When patients known to be infected with HIV are treated differently from others, health care workers may be less aware of the need to adopt appropriate infection control precautions with all patients.

A study of the frequency of needle-stick injuries and blood splashes in Mwanza, Tanzania, found that they were quite common when universal precautions were not in place, with the average health worker being pricked five times and being splashed nine times per year.[5] The annual occupational risk of HIV transmission was estimated at 0.27 percent. This highlights the need for guidelines, training, sharps containers, and supplies of gloves.

Midwives and surgeons are most often at risk, so it is reasonable to train them first. Hospital and clinic workers who look after children are frequently exposed to blood when they insert intravenous drips or take blood samples. Learning to perform these procedures with gloves on takes practice; the gloves need not be sterile and can be washed and reused many times.

Health care workers may also be at risk from other blood-borne viruses, such as hepatitis C and hepatitis B. Practicing universal precautions will protect health care workers from these viruses too.

5. B. Gumodoka et al., "Occupational Exposure to the Risk of HIV Infection among Health Care Workers in Mwanza Region, United Republic of Tanzania," *Bull World Health Organ* 75 (1997): 133–40.

APPROPRIATE DECONTAMINATION METHODS

Level of Risk	Items	Decontamination Method
High risk	Instruments that penetrate the skin or body	Sterilization, or single use of disposables
Moderate risk	Instruments that come in contact with non-intact skin or mucous membrane	Sterilization, boiling, or chemical disinfection
Low risk	Equipment that comes in contact with intact skin	Thorough washing with soap and hot water

Why are they called "universal precautions"?

Many health workers do not understand the term "universal precautions." We call the infection control precautions "universal" because they must be followed with everyone, not just patients known to be infected with HIV. It is not possible to know which patients may be infected with HIV or other blood-borne viruses, so it is essential to adopt the same precautions with all. Sometimes the term "standard precautions" is used in place of "universal precautions."

Is there a risk from mouth-to-mouth resuscitation?

Emergency mouth-to-mouth resuscitation does not carry a risk of transmission of HIV or blood-borne viruses unless there is bleeding from the mouth or face. Where injecting drug use is a problem it is important to remember that when a drug user collapses from an overdose there may be a used needle on that person or nearby.

Can you become infected with HIV from a dead body?

HIV will survive for some hours after the death of an infected patient. However, there is no risk from handling a dead body unless there has been bleeding; gloves should then be worn to clean the body. In addition to the universal precautions already described, anyone performing or assisting in postmortem procedures should wear gloves, masks, protective eyewear, gowns, and waterproof aprons. Instruments and surfaces contaminated during postmortem procedures should be decontaminated with a chemical disinfectant.

How should instruments and surfaces be sterilized to prevent transmission of HIV?[6]

HIV does not survive for long outside the human body. It is sensitive to drying and to heat. Studies show that commonly used chemical disinfectants kill HIV. So the usual methods of sterilizing instruments, equipment, and surfaces will kill HIV, as well as other microorganisms.

Cleaning instruments with soap and water before they are sterilized is essential because viruses can survive chemical disinfection if they are protected within organic matter. Dismantle equipment before cleaning. Select the appropriate method for decontamination according to the guidelines in the table shown above.

Neonatal laryngoscope blades and endotracheal tubes in theaters and delivery rooms are often forgotten. They should be cleaned with surgical spirit, alcohol, or polyvidone iodine after every use.

A solution of sodium hypochlorite (household bleach) in a dilution of 1:10 is an inexpensive and effective disinfectant. However, it must be freshly prepared because it soon becomes inactive. Bleach at 1:10 dilution will corrode metals and plastic so it is best to use a different disinfectant for long-term use for soaking instruments.

---

6. Adapted from WHO, "HIV and the Workplace and Universal Precautions," Fact Sheets for Nurses and Midwives, 2000, *www.who.int/HIV_AIDS/Nursesmidwivesfs/fact-sheet-11*.

UNIVERSAL PRECAUTIONS TO PREVENT TRANSMISSION OF HIV AND OTHER BLOOD-BORNE VIRUSES

These infection control practices should be followed when caring for all patients, at all times:

- Give injections only when absolutely necessary.

- Have a puncture-resistant sharps container close to you when you carry out a procedure using a needle or blade.

- Dispose of used needles immediately in a sharps container. Do not walk around carrying a used needle or blade.

- Never put needles in with general waste.

- Do not re-cap needles or remove them from the syringe after use.

- Wash hands before and after procedures. Cover any sores with a waterproof dressing.

- Do not undertake procedures if you have a weeping or oozing rash.

- Limit skin contact with blood by wearing gloves when putting up intravenous lines or taking blood. Keep sterile gloves for internal examinations and surgical procedures. Change gloves after contact with each patient. Wash hands after removing gloves.

- Use "non-touch" technique for dressings by using forceps.

- Wear a gown or apron for procedures when there might be splashes of blood or body fluids.

- Limit the risk of splashes of blood to mouth or eyes by wearing a mask and goggles for procedures where blood may spurt, e.g., dentistry, surgical operations, and deliveries.

- Use new or sterilized needles, syringes, and instruments for every procedure.

- Mop up spills of blood or other body fluids promptly. Wear gloves while you do this. Then wipe the area with disinfectant.

- Put blood-stained sheets or cloths soiled with blood or body fluids in a plastic bag that will not leak, at the place where they were used. They should be laundered in the usual way.

- Report to the nurse in charge any needle-stick accident, blood splashes to eyes or mouth, or prolonged exposure to blood.

Environmental surfaces such as walls, floors, and other surfaces are not associated with transmission of infections to patients or health care workers. Only ordinary cleaning is necessary and there is no need for fumigation.

How should contaminated waste be handled?

Careful thought should be given to the disposal of sharps containers. They should not be disposed of with general waste because they may end up being a hazard to rag-pickers at waste dumps. If they are buried care should be taken to ensure that they cannot be dug up easily by children playing or by people who may want to "recycle" the needles, such as those who inject drugs. Incineration may be an option.

Place solid waste that is contaminated with blood or body fluids in leak-proof containers and incinerate, or bury it in a deep pit, at least thirty feet away from a water source. Pour liquid waste containing blood or body fluid into a pit latrine or drain connected to an adequately treated sewer.

The De Montfort incinerator is designed to be a relatively cheap unit for disposing of hospital waste. If used correctly it can ensure that waste is exposed to temperatures above 8000° C for a period of over one second. It reduces waste such as dressings, wet or dry, plastics, and organic matter to ash and flue gases. Because needles may not all be reduced to ash care should be taken when removing ashes. Small glass sharps will normally be part melted and rendered safe. The flue gases emitted will have been held at a high temperature for at least one second and should be harmless. There are several designs of different sizes. The Mark 4 is a version specifically designed for use in emergency situations where low cost and a minimum of expensive materials and techniques are priorities. It contains only two metal components and uses firebricks only where these are absolutely necessary. It will burn up to 12 kgs of waste per hour. For further information about these incinerator designs and details of manufacturing the various models apply to Professor D. J. Picken, De Montfort University, Leicester, UK (*djpicken@iee.org.uk*).

How can home-based carers control infection?

Family members and volunteers who help to care for people with AIDS at home can be reassured that there is very little risk of transmission of HIV. Explain to them how to mop up spills of blood or other body fluids. Ideally they should have plastic or rubber gloves, disinfectant, and soap. If gloves are not available, plastic bags can be worn over the hands to avoid contact with blood and body fluids.

What can be done if a health care worker is accidentally exposed to HIV-infected blood?

Immediately following an exposure to blood the health care worker should:

- wash needle-sticks and cuts with soap and water;
- flush splashes to the nose, mouth, or skin with water;
- irrigate eyes with clean water or saline. This should be done gently to avoid harming the eyes.

Using antiseptics, squeezing the wound, or using a caustic agent such as bleach will not reduce the risk of transmission of a blood-borne pathogen and are not recommended.

Should HIV-infected health care workers continue to be employed in health care settings?

There is no reason why health care workers with HIV should have to leave their job, whether or not they became infected through their work, as long as they remain well. Health care workers should be encouraged to reveal their status to a supervisor, who should be obliged to respect their confidentiality. The supervisor should counsel the health care workers about the need to follow universal infection control precautions. The supervisor may be able to protect the health care workers from infectious patients, such as those with tuberculosis or chicken pox. HIV-infected health care workers are in a strong position to provide HIV-related counseling and education, if they are willing. Supervisors should encourage a supportive and nondiscriminatory work environment.

STRATEGIES

Interventions to minimize the risk of transmission of HIV and other blood-borne viruses in health care settings include:

Develop and display guidelines for universal infection control precautions

Detailed local guidelines for precautions, such as the example in the box on page 170, should be prepared and displayed in the treatment room of every clinic and in every ward and theater of the hospital. Most emphasis should be placed on the avoidance of needle-stick injuries, since these are the greatest risk to staff and patients.

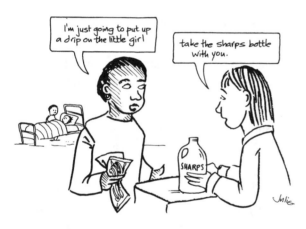

Train health care workers in the use of the guidelines

Traditional healers and traditional birth attendants may be exposed to blood and other body fluids and may use sharps such as blades or needles in their work. They should be included in infection control education.

Supply protective equipment

This includes puncture resistant "sharps" containers, gloves, plastic aprons, gowns and goggles, and disinfectants.

If gloves are difficult to obtain, make sure that they are used for procedures with a greater risk of exposure to blood such as surgery, attending deliveries, suturing, and placing intravenous

cannulae in children. Plastic bags can be used instead of gloves for handling spoiled linen and clearing up spills of blood.

If protective goggles are not available spectacles with clear glass are an inexpensive alternative. Goggles can be made from an old pair of sunglasses or spectacle frames (pop out the lenses). Cut a square of plastic wrap ("cling film") and stretch it over one side of the frame. Hold it taut while someone else applies sticky tape around the rim. Trim the loose edges of the plastic film. Repeat on the other side. These will protect the eyes from splashes during deliveries. But remember that the risk of HIV from eye splashes is very small.

Introduce measures to reduce health workers' stress and fatigue

Stress and fatigue make accidents more likely. Try to ensure appropriate work hours and rosters.

Develop a system for reporting and management of occupational exposures

Those responsible for providing health care services need to document a system to provide adequate assessment, counseling, and follow-up for exposed health care workers. Guidelines and training should include advice to report accidental exposures to blood, and supervisors need to be aware of how to manage such incidents. Refer to staff health policies on post-exposure prophylaxis.

Monitor the implementation of these interventions

ADDITIONAL RESOURCES

Centers for Disease Control and Prevention. "Exposure to Blood — What Health Care Workers Need to Know." CDC, National Center for Infectious Diseases, 1999. *www.cdc.gov/ncidod.*

———. "Updated U.S. Public Health Service Guidelines for the Management of Occupational Exposures to HBV, HCV, and HIV and Recommendations for Post-exposure Prophylaxis," *Morbidity and Mortality Weekly Report* 50, no. RR-11 (2001): 1–52. *www.cdc.gov/hiv/treatment.htm.*

WHO. "HIV and the Workplace and Universal Precautions." Fact sheets for Nurses and Midwives. 2000: *www.who.int.*

GUIDELINES FOR MANAGEMENT OF
ACCIDENTAL EXPOSURE TO HIV-INFECTED BLOOD

- Assess the risk of HIV transmission:

    1. Assess whether the exposure was serious, that is:

        - needle-stick or cut (parenteral)

        - splash to the eye or mouth (mucous-membrane exposure)

        - prolonged skin exposure to large amounts of blood, especially if the skin is broken or inflamed. If there have been only splashes of blood on the skin, then the staff member can be reassured that there is no risk.

    2. Assess the likelihood that the source patient is infected with HIV. Consider:

        - patient's HIV antibody test result if available

        - prevalence of HIV in the population

        - patient's condition

        - possible risk factors of patient

- Inform the source patient of the incident, counsel the individual, request consent to an HIV test.

- If the exposure was serious, and the source patient has AIDS, is positive for HIV antibody, or refuses the test, counsel the health care worker about the risk of infection and the need to practice safe sex. Health care workers should have an HIV test (if they consent) as soon as possible after the exposure. (This will show whether they were already infected with HIV.)

- If after the above assessment there are reasons to think that there may be a risk of transmission of HIV, then the health care worker should be offered the option of post-exposure prophylaxis with a combination of antiretroviral drugs, if they are available.* This should start within twenty-four hours of the exposure and continue for four weeks. Monitoring of side effects will be necessary.

- Advise the health care worker to report and seek medical care if they develop a "flu-like" illness with fever and muscle aches and pains within twelve weeks after the exposure.

- Arrange further HIV tests for the worker six weeks, twelve weeks, and six months after the exposure to determine whether transmission has occurred and arrange follow-up counseling.

- If a health care worker has a needle-stick injury during a surgical operation, there is a small theoretical risk to the patient. The patient should be informed of the incident, and the same procedure outlined above for management of exposures should be followed for both the source health care worker and the exposed patient.

*For recommended regimens and monitoring advice see: Centers for Disease Control and Prevention, "Updated U.S. Public Health Service Guidelines for the Management of Occupational Exposures to HBV, HCV, and HIV and Recommendations for Post-exposure Prophylaxis," *Morbidity and Mortality Weekly Report* 50, no. RR-11 (2001): 1–52. *www.cdc.gov/hiv/treatment.htm.*

SUGGESTED INDICATORS

Indicator	*Method of measurement*
Universal precautions guidelines displayed in health care settings and available to home-based care staff and volunteers	Observation
Safe sharps container available and in use in health care settings	Observation
Gloves available and in use for procedures involving exposure to blood	Observation
Proportion of health care staff trained in use of universal precautions guidelines	Training records
Proportion of procedures undertaken according to the guidelines	Observation of a sample of procedures using a checklist
System for reporting needle-stick incidents in place	Up-to-date register of needle-stick incidents
Management protocol for needle-stick incidents available	Observation
Proportion of supervisors and senior staff aware of management protocol for needle-stick incidents	Interview survey of supervisors or senior staff
Proportion of reported needle-stick injuries adequately followed up	Review of records/anonymous survey of health care workers
Satisfaction of HIV-infected patients that they are being treated in a nondiscriminatory way	Focus group discussions with PLWH group.

14

Providing Care and Support

Billy Mosedame of Botswana, a man living with HIV, declared at an international conference on home-based care: "We all need and deserve care, support, and compassion." Nondiscriminatory health care is a human right.

The following story was told during an evaluation of an HIV-prevention project:

The mother of a young man who was ill with HIV had spent a lot of money on medicines that had not worked. But when she discovered that her son had AIDS the family lifted the ill boy on his bedding and left him by the side of the road. No one would touch him. Project staff came and helped the boy and took him to the hospital, where he was treated and made a good recovery. Meanwhile the project staff talked with his family and gave them information about how HIV does and does not spread and encouraged the family to accept their son back into the family. Because the family saw the staff were not afraid to touch and care for their son they felt ashamed, changed their attitude, and welcomed him back. The family were grateful to the project staff for their intervention. The neighbors also asked questions about how HIV spreads.

This is a very important story. It demonstrates how successfully attitudes can be changed and shows the connection between care and prevention. When families are reassured about how HIV does not spread and see others touching people with HIV, then they are more willing to accept HIV-positive family members. Others are also then less likely to discriminate against positive people. When people see that they will not be discriminated against, they are more likely to be willing to come forward for testing, counseling, and treatment, and to make efforts to ensure that they do not transmit the infection

to others. It becomes possible for them to lead productive positive lives. Also when local families see that neighbors are affected by HIV, they are more likely to believe that it is possible for them to be affected too and to become interested to learn how the virus spreads so that they can protect themselves.

Prevention efforts that begin with care and support are more likely to be effective and less likely to increase stigmatization than attempts to change behavior through information and education approaches alone.

At present, there is no cure for AIDS. However, there are treatments for the relief of symptoms, medicines to treat and prevent opportunistic infections, and an increasing range of antiretroviral drugs that attack HIV itself.

To meet the physical, emotional, social, and economic needs of PLWH, care and support should be governed by the same principles as those described on page 55. In particular ethical issues need to be considered, including the importance of informed consent to treatment, respect for dignity, privacy, and confidentiality, quality of care, equality of access, affordability, effectiveness, and efficiency.

Appropriate care and support for people living with HIV will enable them to live longer, healthier, and more productive lives, which benefits the individuals, their families, and the whole society.

RATIONALE

The continuum of care

Voluntary counseling and testing should be an entry point to a continuum of care. Sometimes people will be well for years after they learn their HIV status. Others may learn that they have HIV only when they contract a serious opportunistic infection or malignancy.

THE HIV/AIDS CONTINUUM OF CARE

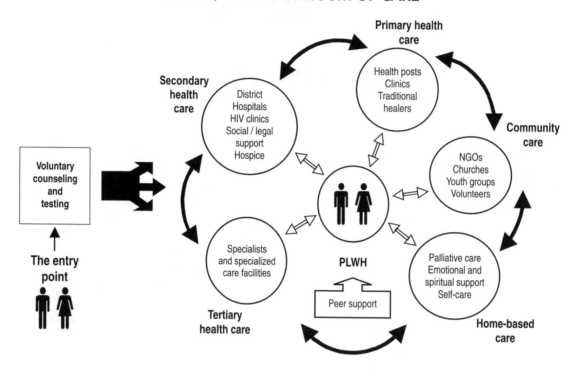

Source: D. Miller, *Key Elements in HIV/AIDS Care and Support,* WHO/UNAIDS, September 2000

Ideally, even in humanitarian settings, people with HIV-related illness would be able to be cared for in their own home or shelter, with support from their family, friends, and community. Their symptoms and signs should be assessed by health workers at the local clinic, or by outreach health workers, and if they need to be hospitalized, there should be trained nurses and doctors, appropriate standard treatment protocols, and essential drugs available to treat the most common opportunistic infections. The idea of a continuum of care is that there will be links between the hospital, clinics, community care, and home-based care, so that people do not get discharged from the hospital without any support and are able to be referred to specialist services from a primary health care clinic.

The ideal of a continuum of care can be achieved only with much consultation, communication, and coordination, between a range of stakeholders who provide care in these different settings. Even in humanitarian settings it is important to develop links between the levels of care that may be available.

Home-based care and self-care

When PLWH are able to accept their diagnosis, they often start to live in a healthier way. They may give up smoking cigarettes, drinking, or injecting drugs. They may try to improve their diet, take regular exercise, and reduce their levels of stress. All this will help to prevent infections that may further damage their immune system and may restore a sense of control.

Once a PLWH becomes sick, experience in many countries shows that home-based care is often appropriate and acceptable. Most patients prefer to be looked after at home. Even in humanitarian settings people may prefer to be cared for in their own shelter by family members rather than in a hospital. Where HIV is common, home-based care may be the only way to care for the large numbers of patients when hospital services are overwhelmed.

Home-based care requires training, support, supervision, and equipment. A hospital may deploy an outreach team that undertakes home visits. More commonly a team of volunteers is trained to provide care and support. It is important that carers know that they can refer patients to the clinic or hospital when necessary. Discharge policies need to be in place to ensure that arrangements are coordinated for home-based care before the patient is discharged from the hospital. Caring for patients with AIDS is stressful. Volunteers must be treated with the same respect as health professionals. We also need to recognize that the burden of home-based care generally falls disproportionately on women. Childcare and preparing for the future care of orphaned children are important components of home-based care programs.

When a PLWH receives care visits, the family and neighbors know that the patient has AIDS. The visits raise awareness of AIDS in the community. This can lead to useful community discussion about the need for behavior change.[1] Experience has shown that there is a strong link between home care and community action to prevent spread of HIV.

Nutritional support

IEC materials about nutrition should be prepared in consultation with PLWH and their carers to ensure that the advice given is feasible, with appropriate foods and methods of preparation.

People with HIV who are asymptomatic should try to eat a variety of foods with sufficient calories and micronutrients. It is especially important that pregnant women infected with HIV have a good diet, with sufficient calories and plenty of fruits and vegetable, to maintain their health and reduce the risk that HIV will pass to the baby.

PLWH often have a poor appetite. They may have frequent diarrhea and vomiting. PLWH who are ill may feel better if they can eat frequent small meals. Soft foods, such as soups and mashed bananas, are easier to eat for those who have an inflamed throat. Many societies have fermented foods or drinks, either dairy-based (such as yogurt) or cereal-based (such as mahewu). Fermentation increases the digestibility of foods, increases the absorption of micronutrients, and decreases bacterial contamination. Those who are too ill to eat may need to be fed via a naso-gastric tube. It would be unusual to manage this at home in humanitarian settings but may be possible with support, depending on the context.

Exercise

There is evidence that stress is harmful to the immune system and may make HIV disease progress more quickly. Relaxation exercises, including progressive muscle relaxation, meditation, and massage, can help people with HIV to cope and lessen feelings of anxiety and depression.

Other exercise, including walking and running, can also be beneficial to people living with HIV. Certain exercises can strengthen leg muscles, which may become weak in patients with HIV-related symptoms.

Home nursing care

Weight loss, fever, night sweats, diarrhea, and itchy skin disorders are common early symptoms and signs of HIV infection. Good nursing care such as washing, frequent mouth washes, and massage can be a great help to patients. Nursing care needs to include sympathetic psychological support for patients who may often feel frightened. There are a number of simple medicines that can relieve symptoms:

- chlorpheniramine for itching and drug reactions
- calamine lotion for itchy rashes
- prochlorperazine for vomiting
- oral rehydration fluids for diarrhea
- analgesics, such as aspirin or acetaminophen (paracetamol) for pain
- aspirin or acetaminophen (paracetamol) for fever
- loperamide for diarrhea

There may be traditional remedies that will also relieve symptoms.

1. C. M. Chela, I. D. Campbell, and Z. Siankanga, "Clinical Care as Part of Integrated AIDS Management in a Zambian Rural Community," *AIDS Care* 1 (1989): 319–25.

Palliative care[2]

Palliative care is the care of someone who cannot be cured and who is too sick for carers to be able to prolong their life. Palliative care enables people to die with dignity. Palliative care does not hasten or try to postpone death. It aims to provide relief from pain and distressing symptoms and spiritual and psychological support to the patient and the patient's family as they prepare for death.

Carers often find it difficult to talk with people who are dying and to express the love and compassion that they feel. For carers who are HIV positive themselves dealing with death can be especially difficult because of their own fears.

Even in cultures where it is not traditional to talk about death, people who are dying are usually grateful for the opportunity to talk about it. It is important to help PLWH to arrange for the care of their children after their death and to prepare their children for their death. Often the stigma associated with AIDS prevents parents from telling their children what is going on, and this contributes to the confusion and grief that children feel when their parents die. PLWH may also need help to prepare a will or may need legal advice to prevent problems when their assets are distributed after their death.

Common physical symptoms in the final stages of AIDS are

- cough
- diarrhea
- loss of appetite and wasting
- itching
- weakness and fatigue
- fever
- difficulty swallowing
- psychiatric symptoms — anxiety, depression, agitation
- pain

Effective management of pain is one of the most important components of palliative care. It is likely to be difficult to achieve in many humanitarian settings because export/import controls may make it difficult to obtain supplies of controlled drugs such as diazepam and morphine. Drug control authorities in the receiving country may not be functioning or may not have authority for the refugee- and IDP-affected areas. This is why humanitarian aid agencies do not provide narcotics in their emergency medical supplies. This difficulty has been recognized and is being addressed by WHO and the International Narcotics Control Board (INCB). The INCB and the Forty-Ninth World Health Assembly have recommended that control obligations be limited to the authorities of exporting countries in emergency situations. Model guidelines have been prepared to assist national authorities with simplified regulatory procedures. The guidelines and a model shipment request form are provided in the New Emergency Health Kit (WHO).[3] This may help in negotiations with the appropriate national drug control authorities to be able to obtain the opiate drugs needed for palliative care.

Pain may result from local tissue damage to skin or organs, or may result from pressure on or destruction of nerves. Pain also has an emotional component: when people are feeling low they may experience pain as more severe than when they are feeling happier, or perhaps distracted by a visiting friend.

The individuals feeling the pain need to make the decisions about pain relief. This is because they alone experience their symptoms, and also because a sense of control is very important at this stage of an illness.

The first step is simple analgesics, such as aspirin and acetaminophen (paracetamol), and good nursing care to ensure that the patient is as comfortable as possible. For example a simple soothing cream may be applied to inflamed rashes or the anal area.

When these measures become ineffective, weak opioid drugs such as codeine, combined with either aspirin or acetaminophen (paracetamol), will be required, although they may be difficult to obtain in some humanitarian settings. These tablets may cause constipation.

2. UNAIDS, *Palliative Care*, UNAIDS Technical Update, October 2000.

3. *The New Emergency Health Kit* (Geneva: WHO, 1998).

The third step requires stronger painkillers in the form of strong opioid drugs. WHO's New Emergency Health Kit (1998) includes morphine injection, whereas the previous UNHCR essential drug list included pentazocine injection, which is inferior but may be a practical alternative when opioids are not available.[4] Morphine, taken by mouth as syrup or tablets, is the most effective drug for palliative care. It needs to be given every four hours, and regularly, in order to prevent the pain from returning, rather than waiting until pain returns. Injections of morphine (under the skin) should be used only when the patient cannot swallow. Intramuscular injections are painful, especially when the patient has reduced muscle mass.

The side effects of morphine are:

• constipation (which may be beneficial when the patient has diarrhea),

• nausea and vomiting (antinausea treatment can be given),

• drowsiness, which wears off over time, and

• dry mouth (the patient will need frequent sips of water)

There is no need to worry that the patient may become addicted to the drug; the important aim is pain relief. However, it is not always legal to give morphine to these patients, even when it is available. We should advocate strongly that morphine be available to patients dying from AIDS-related illnesses.

Other medicines that may be helpful include tricyclic antidepressants for nerve pain, steroids, anticonvulsants, and antispasmodics.

Restlessness that sometimes accompanies dying may be relieved by diazepam, which can be given via the rectum if the patient cannot take it by mouth. Check first for possible treatable causes of the restlessness such as urinary retention or pain.

---

4. WHO New Emergency Health Kit: "Pentazocine and tramadol, Diazepam and phenobarbitol are now controlled drugs in some countries and come under control measure additional to the UN Convention on Psychotropic Substances, resulting in the requirement for an import permit before authorization of an export permit."

Respite care

Respite care is temporary care that enables the usual carer to have a rest from the stress and work of caring for an ill person. When respite care is available, family and friends are more willing to care for PLWH and are able to have a better relationship with the person. The morale of both the patient and the carer will be improved. Respite care might be provided through a day-care center, a residential center, a drop-in center — or as respite for carers in their own home. Provision of regular and reliable respite care should be a priority for home-based care programs. There should be a clear time limit. Respite care might be provided through a roster of volunteers. This may be difficult to arrange in humanitarian settings, and respite care in the hospital may be the only option.

Primary health care

The skills, knowledge, and supplies to support home- and community-based care need to be available at the primary health care level. The primary health care clinic should be the contact point for referral to hospital care and other relevant services.

Management of opportunistic infections

There is a wide range of clinical manifestations associated with HIV infection. We do not know the cause of all of them. Some are due to a direct effect of the virus on certain body cells, such as those of the central nervous system and gastrointestinal tract. But many clinical manifestations are the result of damage to the immune system, which leaves the body open to infection by a variety of opportunistic organisms. Infections that are latent in the body, such as tuberculosis or herpes zoster, reactivate when immunity weakens. The most common infections suffered by people living with HIV are tuberculosis, pneumonia, diarrhea, candida infection of the mouth and throat, STIs, and fungal skin infections. These infections can often be diagnosed at primary health care clinics and generally respond to affordable antibiotics. Gynecological problems are common in women infected with HIV. Most women prefer to be seen by a female health worker and want to be examined in privacy. There is a need for resource materials about HIV-related illnesses in local languages.

Prophylaxis

Prophylaxis means taking a medicine to prevent rather than treat an infection. Studies show that the antibiotic co-trimoxazole can prevent many bacterial and parasitic opportunistic infections in adults and children living with HIV, including toxoplasmosis, salmonellosis, pneumococcal pneumonia, and bacteremia. This is a cost-effective intervention for people living with HIV and governments because it reduces hospital admissions and mortality.

WHO recommends that all HIV-infected adults with symptomatic disease and asymptomatic individuals with a CD4 count of less than 500 (see page 182 for a definition of the CD4 count) should take a daily double-strength dose of co-trimoxazole (trimethoprim 160 mg; sulfamethoxazole 800 mg). Pregnant women infected with HIV should take co-trimoxazole only after the first trimester. The infants of HIV-positive mothers should also receive co-trimoxazole syrup from six weeks of age, as should any child identified as being infected with HIV during the first year of life and children older than fifteen months who have symptoms of HIV infection.

This prophylaxis should continue indefinitely unless there are side effects. If severe skin rashes occur the co-trimoxazole should be stopped. Patients will need to be followed up every month initially and then every three months.

Isoniazid prophylaxis is recommended for people living with HIV at risk of tuberculosis, such as those with a positive TB skin test or who are living in areas where the disease is endemic. Isoniazid has been shown to increase the survival of HIV-infected persons at risk of tuberculosis. Since isoniazid is relatively inexpensive, this is likely to be a cost-effective measure, especially in the high-risk setting of refugee and IDP camps, where tuberculosis can spread easily.

Detection and management of tuberculosis

In many countries where conflict leads to displacement, tuberculosis (TB) is the most common opportunistic infection in people living with HIV and the most common cause of death. Tuberculosis may occur at any stage in the course of immunodeficiency. TB control programs should be integrated with primary health care services for the displaced and conflict-affected population.

WHO has prepared a field manual on tuberculosis control in refugee/IDP settings.[5] It is recommended that a TB control program should not begin until crude mortality rates have been reduced to less than 1 per 10,000 population per day, basic needs are provided, and essential clinical services and supplies are available.

Because tuberculosis requires a long duration of treatment and there is a risk of resistant organisms developing if the course of treatment is not followed, a TB control program should be implemented only if the security situation is stable and the camp population is expected to remain for at least six months. Funding should be available for at least twelve months, along with sufficient medical supplies and trained staff.

The national TB program of the host country should be involved in the implementation of a TB program for the displaced population.

The priority of a TB control program is to identify and treat infectious patients and ensure that they become noninfectious as soon as possible. Successful cure of infectious patients will reduce transmission. If drugs are taken regularly patients become noninfectious within two weeks of beginning the treatment.

In addition to the infectious smear-positive pulmonary TB patients, severely ill patients with nonpulmonary TB (who are not generally infectious) should be treated in the TB program. People with noninfectious TB who are not severely ill need not be included in the TB program until it has been demonstrated that cure rates are satisfactory.

5. WHO, *Tuberculosis Control in Refugee Situations: An Inter-Agency Field Manual* (1997).

People living with HIV who have tuberculosis respond well to standard TB treatment. The recommended strategy for curing infectious TB patients is the WHO TB control strategy: Directly Observed Therapy Short course, or DOTS. This is implemented by providing the correct combination of TB drugs for six or eight months and observing patients swallowing their medicines. This is especially important during the first two months of treatment.

TB is a wasting disease. Many displaced persons may also be suffering from malnutrition. TB treatment will usually lead to an increased need for calories; therefore attention to nutrition will be an important component of a TB control program in humanitarian situations.

Supportive counseling

The availability of well-informed, nonjudgmental, and objective supportive counseling can assist people infected with and affected by HIV to live useful and productive lives (see chapter 7).

Health care consultations provide an opportunity to give information and to talk about prevention. People living with HIV may also need good advice about and access to methods of contraception.

Those who inject drugs need well-informed advice and support. They may need referral to drug substitution and rehabilitation services if these are available. If they continue to inject it is essential to provide supplies of needles and syringes in order to protect others and to counsel them about the need for safe sex.

The role of traditional healers

In many of the countries severely affected by HIV, people often have recourse to traditional healers when ill and respect their knowledge and power to heal. There are many examples of traditional or spiritual healers and modern health practitioners working together in HIV prevention and care. Traditional healers have been trained to recognize and counsel HIV-infected patients. When the traditional healer gives the same prevention advice as hospital or clinic staff, the message is likely to be very effective. Traditional healers may also be able to provide important relief for HIV-related symptoms.

Referral system

It is important that staff at the primary health care level know when and how to refer patients for further investigation or treatment. Standard treatment protocols for common problems in people living with HIV need to include indications for referral. It is helpful for PHC-level staff to receive feedback from the hospital about the appropriateness of their referral and the outcome. But even where referral systems are in place, they are often not used. It is necessary to monitor whether systems are followed at the hospital level. Problems with communications and transport are often obstacles to effective referral. Intersectoral and community consultation are necessary to identify solutions to these problems.

Hospital care

The opportunistic infections suffered by PLWH generally respond well to treatment but tend to recur frequently. This means that adults and children with HIV may require frequent admission to the hospital. It is helpful to keep their notes on the ward and to try to make their admissions as brief and as comfortable as possible. Studies have found that lack of information about the patient's condition and progress adds to the stress of family members. Patients with HIV do not need to be isolated unless there are patients in the ward with infections that PLWH may be susceptible to, such as chickenpox or hepatitis. The need for guidelines on universal infection control precautions is described in chapter 13.

Diagnosis and staging of HIV disease

The combination of symptoms and signs of advanced HIV disease means that it is generally not difficult to diagnose clinically; however, HIV-negative tuberculosis may have a similar clinical presentation. It is desirable to be able to test patients who are suspected on clinical grounds to have HIV infection. Patients should always be counseled before and after testing. There is no need to test patients who are unconscious or otherwise unable to give informed consent. Policies on testing patients and arrangements to keep results confidential need to be discussed and documented. An alphabetical code system can be used to avoid labeling specimens and results with patient's names. The strategy for confirmation of HIV tests for diagnosis is outlined in appendix B (page 199).

WHO categorizes clinical status into four stages, which indicate the level of immune suppression and the prognosis of people living with HIV:

- Stage 1: asymptomatic infection.

- Stage 2: early (mild) disease.

- Stage 3: intermediate (moderate) disease.

- Stage 4: late (severe) disease.

The "CD4 count" refers to the number of CD4 white cells in the blood. These are the white cells that control the immune system and are most affected by HIV. This laboratory test is not widely available. The total white cell count also drops in immune deficiency — but is a less useful marker. Manifestations of HIV disease are rare at CD4 counts above 500×10^6 cells/l and severe illness and death are rare in patients with counts above 200×10^6/l.

Bacterial infection of the blood can require admission to the hospital. Gram-negative organisms are the most common cause of infection, especially nontyphoid Salmonella species. Pneumococcal pneumonia, meningitis, and septicemia are also frequent and may occur earlier than Gram-negative infections. Many people with AIDS suffer severe wasting, with chronic diarrhea and fever. Poor appetite and reduced food intake contribute to the wasting. A variety of protozoal and bacterial infections may cause diarrhea but often no specific cause can be found.

AIDS can present with florid pulmonary tuberculosis. The X-ray appearances are often atypical with the middle or lower lobes more commonly affected and the upper lobes often clear. Enlargement of hilar lymph nodes and effusions are common. Mycobacteria may disseminate through the body, causing miliary tuberculosis or meningitis. Tuberculous lymphadenopathy is common.

Skin manifestations may be due to neoplastic disease, especially Kaposi sarcoma, or they may be of an inflammatory nature. These include drug reactions, infections such as secondary syphilis, seborrheic dermatitis, and psoriasis. Generalized dry skin is a common problem in HIV infection. It is often very itchy.

Neurological disease is also a common cause for admission. HIV can infect cells in the central nervous system (CNS) and cause neurological problems. The CNS may also be affected by opportunistic infections and tumors. Cerebral toxoplasmosis (presenting as a space occupying lesion of the brain) and cryptococcal meningitis (presenting as chronic meningitis) are the most common infections. Neurological manifestations usually occur late in the course of HIV infection. Dementia is the most common problem, but almost any neurological symptoms may occur. Psychiatric disorders may be confused with neurological disease. Organic and psychiatric diseases often occur together.

In resource-poor settings it can be difficult to identify different opportunistic infections without access to specific laboratory tests. There are a number of manuals and slide sets that can be helpful in training health care staff to recognize the signs of common HIV-related opportunistic infections and cancers. Standard treatment protocols need to be developed for cost-effective management of the common problems that affect people infected with HIV.

Antiretroviral treatment

Antiretroviral drugs (ARVs) kill HIV and so reduce the level of virus in the blood. A combination of these drugs needs to be taken for life, and they often have side effects. PLWH who are able to access these drugs can remain well for many years, although the virus remains in the body. However, despite recent price reductions these drugs remain out of reach for most PLWH. In recent years pilot programs have shown that it is possible to increase access to ARVs even in resource-poor settings.

There are three classes of drugs that prevent HIV from multiplying by blocking the action of viral enzymes, but they do not remove the virus from the body. They are the nucleoside reverse transcriptase inhibitors (NRTIs), nonnucleoside reverse transcriptase inhibitors (NNRTIs), and the protease inhibitors (PIs). Because HIV mutates rapidly within the body it becomes resistant to drugs, so ARVs need to be used in expensive combinations. Guidelines for treatment of HIV recommend lifelong triple therapy, commonly two NRTIs, combined with a PI or NNRTI.[6] These combinations are called "highly active antiretroviral therapy" (HAART). Specialists have to monitor the patient's viral load, blood cells, and liver and renal function because of side effects. For the drugs to be effective the person has to take them correctly at least 95 percent of the time, and they have to be taken for life. Some are not able to tolerate the side effects.

Experts disagree about how early to start treatment. Some believe that it is best to wait until the patient's white cell count falls below $500 \times 10^6/l$, or the patient develops symptoms. Others think that treatment should begin even when the patient is asymptomatic. However, the long-term side effects of these drugs are not known; early use might limit later use of the drugs; use by people without symptoms turns them into patients; long-term compliance is likely to be poor; and treatment is costly.

Drugs and medical supplies

There may be a need to add new items to essential drugs lists, such as nevirapine for prevention of mother-to-child transmission of HIV and drugs to treat specific opportunistic infections, taking into account national drug policies and costs. In addition it is important to ensure adequate supplies of the antibiotics and antifungal drugs needed to treat common HIV-related conditions and analgesics and other medicines essential for palliative care. Adequate quantities of condoms, gloves, needles, syringes, and surgical equipment also need to be obtained.

Discharge policy

It is important that mechanisms are established to ensure continuity of care when patients are discharged. Home-based care has rarely been implemented in humanitarian settings so this will be a challenge. Family members need good information about the patient's needs and the likely outcome, with the consent of the patient. Local primary health care staff and a home-based care service if available should be informed of the discharge and given details of necessary follow-up care. Efficient discharge and referral policies are cost-effective because well-informed and motivated carers can reduce the need for readmission.

The following aspects of patient's needs should be assessed before discharge:

- psychological and neurological problems such as agitation, difficulty in concentrating, and disturbances in sleeping and eating patterns;
- degree of disability and potential future disabilities;
- psychosocial problems (social isolation, anxiety, anger, blame, guilt);
- physical care needs;
- need for pain management;
- the greatest concerns expressed by the client or patient.

Care and support for orphans

The effects on children in a family affected by AIDS begin long before the parents die. Decreased income or productivity when the breadwinner becomes ill and spending on medicines and health care services result in the family's assets being depleted. Children suffer the emotional effects of seeing their parents die slowly from an often painful illness. They may be the only ones who care for their parents and may miss school. They may be stigmatized by neighbors, teachers, and schoolchildren.

Because of stigma, parents may be reluctant to tell their children about their diagnosis. The Memory Books Programme in Uganda aims to support HIV-positive mothers to tell their children of their serostatus.[7] Mother and children write the memory book together and record important family history. Parents are encouraged to take time preparing the memory books

6. WHO, "Scaling Up Antiretroviral Therapy in Resource-Limited Settings: Guidelines for a Public Health Approach" (Geneva: WHO, April 2002).

7. "The Dilemma of HIV-Positive Parents Revealing Serostatus to Their Children," *Nyamayarwo* (2000), MoOrD250.

🎗 DISCUSSION POINT 🎗

Until recently the cost of lifelong treatment with a combination of ARVs put it out of reach for all but a small elite in developing countries. We could describe these drugs simply as "not available." However, persistent advocacy efforts and pressures created by generic drug companies in some developing countries have led to dramatic reductions in prices. A year's supply of medication may now cost only a few hundred dollars. Where HIV infection is not yet common it should be possible even in developing countries to encourage identification of those infected with the assurance that they will receive treatment. However, where prevalence is high it will not be possible to treat everyone.

The cheaper price of ARVs and the development of simpler regimens with three drugs combined in a single tablet raise questions for those responsible for health care services in refugee/IDP settings.

- Refugee/IDP settings are unpredictable. What will happen if refugees/IDPs start a course of lifelong treatment, requiring monitoring, but then travel home or are transferred to another camp at short notice?

- Incorrect use of the drugs can lead to resistance. How could we increase the likelihood that drugs are taken in correct dosage and long-term?

- Because of the controlled environment it may be easier to implement an ARV program in a refugee/IDP camp than in the local host population. How could this inequality be avoided?

- What are some of the barriers to providing treatment in refugee/IDP settings? How can we best prepare for reductions in prices of drugs?

The drugs are not the only cost of providing effective treatment. There are also the costs of follow up, laboratory monitoring tests, and training of doctors and nurses. Trials will be needed to determine cost-effective regimens that minimize the risk of development of drug resistance and maximize continuity of treatment, monitoring systems, and protocols for treatment failures. Where treatment programs for tuberculosis are in place these offer an opportunity to integrate treatment of HIV with antiretrovirals. The provision of ARVs in refugee/IDP settings needs to be considered in the light of national policy.

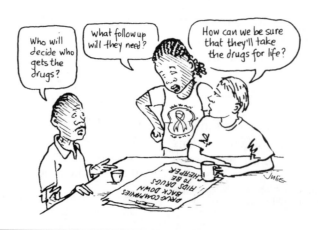

☙ DISCUSSION POINT ☙

What information should be recorded on outpatient cards? These cards are essential for communication between health care workers who may see a patient on different occasions. It is necessary to communicate the fact that the patient has been tested for HIV and whether or not the patient has been counseled. However, if information on HIV status is recorded on patient-held records, the patient is at risk of exposure of his or her HIV status. Could symbols or codes be used to record: "blood taken for HIV antibody test," "HIV antibody positive," and "counseled about HIV infection"? Could a separate card be used for information about HIV? Would any of these methods succeed for long, or would the public soon learn about them?

---

because they include the sensitive issues of loss and changes ahead.

After the death of one or both parents children may suffer many changes in caregivers and repeated bereavements. Orphaned children often undertake tasks that are beyond the level of responsibility usual at their age — for example, a twelve-year-old girl may be left to care for siblings. Their education is often compromised because they need to stay at home to care for others or to work, or because of lack of school fees. This reduces their opportunities for future employment. Poverty is an almost inevitable result of being orphaned. This adds to stigmatization and increases vulnerability to exploitation. Orphans may undertake hazardous activities to support themselves, including sex work.

The health status of orphaned children is often poor. Mothers are the most important providers of primary health care; they recognize when their child is ill and provide comfort and extra attention that may avert more serious illness. They are often the recipients of health promotion information such as oral rehydration procedures for diarrhea and the benefits of vaccination. Grandparents and siblings may be less able to provide such care.

The loss of parents has an intergenerational impact. Children who lack parental love and support and a sense of belonging to family and community often grow up with psychological problems and may experience difficulties in their adult relationships and in parenting their own children.

There is therefore an urgent need to arrange for appropriate care and support for orphaned children, no matter what the cause of their orphan status. Support for orphans and other children in need should be integrated into the community's response to the need for home-based care.

The primary aim is to try to keep orphaned children within their own extended family. Families may need assistance to enable them to care for orphans. If this is not possible, then children should be cared for in a foster family, preferably within their own community. Studies have shown that orphanages are not an ideal environment for children and are expensive. Institutional care often harms the emotional health of children and means that they lose links with their own communities and their sense of belonging. They leave the orphanage when they are still very young adults and have to make their way in the world without any support from relatives or friends.

In humanitarian settings the conflict that led to displacement may have led to large numbers of orphaned or unaccompanied children requiring care within their extended families or with foster parents. In places where HIV is common there will also be large numbers of orphaned children. This can result in the coping mechanisms of the community becoming overwhelmed. There will be increasing numbers of households headed by children or by elderly grandparents. Financial and practical support will need to be provided to affected households to enable them to care for increased numbers of children.

STRATEGIES

Prioritize care and support activities

Care and support activities can be described at three levels of complexity and cost.[8]

1. Essential activities

   - HIV voluntary counseling and testing;

   - psychosocial support for PLWH and their families;

   - palliative care;

   - treatment for common opportunistic infections;

   - nutritional care;

   - STI care and family planning services;

   - co-trimoxazole prophylaxis;

   - reduction of stigma and discrimination.

2. Activities of intermediate complexity and cost. In addition to the above:

   - active case finding and treatment for TB; prophylaxis for TB;

   - systemic antifungal agents for severe fungal infections;

   - treatment for HIV-associated malignancies: Kaposi's sarcoma, lymphoma, and cervical cancer;

   - treatment for herpes simplex and herpes zoster infections;

   - antiretroviral prophylaxis to prevent mother-to-child transmission of HIV;

   - post-exposure prophylaxis following rape, and occupational exposure;

   - funding of community efforts that reduce the impact of HIV.

3. Activities of high complexity and cost. In addition to the above:

   - highly active antiretroviral therapy;

   - diagnosis and treatment of opportunistic infections that are difficult to diagnose and/or expensive to treat, such as atypical mycobacterial infections, cytomegalovirus infection, multiresistant TB, and toxoplasmosis;

   - specific public welfare services that reduce the economic and social impacts.

In the post-emergency phase in humanitarian settings it should be possible to provide at least the essential care and support activities. The choice of strategies will depend on the prevalence of HIV in the refugee or IDP population and the stage of the epidemic. If there are very few people ill with HIV they represent little additional burden to health care services and it is relatively easy to provide support to those who care for the PLWH at home and in the community. However, when HIV is common and many people are sick and dying, the capacity of the community to respond with home-based care and support for orphans is reduced. Good coordination of care and support is essential.

Develop policies

Policies and protocols need to be developed appropriate for each level of health care service delivery. It will be helpful to establish a small committee with representatives of people living with HIV, refugees/IDPs, health staff, administration, appropriate NGOs, and host health officials to formulate these policies. Policies should be consistent with national guidelines.

Policies will need to be developed to address:

- HIV testing for diagnosis (ensuring confidentiality);

- prevention of discrimination and stigma against PLWH in health settings;

- treatment or management protocols for common HIV-related conditions;

- referral protocols and discharge co-ordination;

- universal precautions for infection control.

8. WHO/UNAIDS, "Key Elements in HIV/AIDS Care and Support," September 2000, *www.unaids.org*.

PLWH-FRIENDLY HOSPITALS

The idea of accrediting hospitals that are "friendly" to PLWH is being studied in India, based on the model of "baby-friendly hospitals" that fulfill criteria supportive of breast-feeding. A set of indicators has been developed that include: (1) HIV testing voluntary, confidential, and accompanied by pre- and post-test counseling; universal precautions practiced with all patients; information about HIV status kept confidential; people with HIV not segregated; (2) staff trained in the basics of HIV/AIDS and transmission; clinical staff trained in case management; staff trained on rights and needs of HIV-positive people; (3) trained counselors available for additional counseling; systems for referral and follow-up in place for other sources of care and support.

—Gilborn, Population Council, study currently under way in India, 2001.

Train health care staff

Health care staff at all levels require training in the management and nursing care of adults and children infected with HIV, and in referral and discharge processes.

The need for confidentiality, and mechanisms to ensure this, need to be discussed with mortuary attendants, clerks, porters, general hands, and drivers as well as doctors, nurses, and health workers.

All categories of staff will also need information and reassurance about the risk of occupational exposure to HIV (see page 167).

Establish home-based care system

The way that home-based care is organized will vary from one setting to another. It is important that communities identify their own needs and participate fully in the development of a system. Populations that have been displaced, whether they are living in camps or in resettled areas, have usually experienced a breakdown in their community structures and networks. In this context a home-based care system may rely on care from family members, with support from health care workers at the nearest health care facility. However, community structures that may be able to coordinate teams of home-care volunteers, such as church or faith-based organizations, traditional chiefs, and elected representatives, may still be in place. These community groups may have different agendas and constituencies; the relationships between community structures need to be taken into account to avoid tensions. Before planning it is important to find out whether there is already any organized support for home-based care — for example, by church groups.

The following are important components of a home-based care system:

- recruitment, training, and ongoing support for volunteers;

- identification of households in need of support and assessment of their care needs;

- distribution of home-based care kits (see the following page for kit contents);

- guidelines for home-based care volunteers or carers for nursing care, infection control, and waste management;

- distribution system for supplies for home-based care;

- supportive visits, including spiritual support;

- access to legal advice in relation to writing wills;

- coordination with nearest health care facility and respite care.

People living with HIV may play an important role as volunteer carers for others with HIV-related illness. People with HIV-related disease are often young and may prefer to be cared for by their peers. Young people are often willing to become involved in home-based care work.

Family carers are often women who are already looking after children or elderly dependents; some family carers may be elderly or very young; often family carers may themselves be living with HIV.

Caring for people with chronic illness at home is very stressful. It is very important that carers are able to access respite care and counseling. Home-based care is cost-effective and saves the health care system money. It is often appropriate to provide an incentive or small allowance to home-based care volunteers. This should be discussed with the community, and thought should be given to sustainability.

Home-based care kits help volunteers to look after the sick person well and safely. Such kits might contain:

- analgesics, antibiotics, and antifungal medicines;
- antiseptics;
- emollient cream;
- vitamin and mineral supplements;
- disposable diapers, bandages, aprons, and gloves.

Arrange care and support for carers

Health care professionals are used to being able to cure their patients especially children. However, when the illness is caused by HIV, patients relapse frequently, and health care workers often come to know the patient and their parents well by the time the patient dies. Health care workers are likely to be working hard and have little time to grieve with the family. This inability to cure their patients, and the sadness that they witness and share are stressful and upsetting for health care workers at all levels.

Health care work in humanitarian settings is always stressful, with scarce resources, poor facilities, and high rates of infectious disease caused by overcrowding and poor nutritional status. Where HIV is common the workload in clinics and hospitals is further increased.

Caregivers, whether health care professionals, home-based care volunteers, or relatives, may experience stigma and discrimination because they look after PLWH. The caregivers themselves may be infected with HIV, or at risk of infection with HIV, and may have to cope with their own fears of becoming ill, dependent, and dying. They are members of the community and may be coping with multiple bereavements following the loss of friends and family members.

For all these reasons managers need to provide opportunities for health care staff and volunteers to meet and discuss their fears and concerns and to receive confidential counseling if needed. Care needs to be taken to minimize stress in the workplace and to try to avoid excessive workload being placed on too few staff.

Coordinate care and support for orphans and other dependents

It is likely to be more straightforward to support community efforts to respond to the needs raised by the HIV epidemic in stable communities than in humanitarian settings. Where people have been displaced it may be especially difficult to arrange appropriate care for children who have been orphaned, whether because of HIV infection, other illnesses, or violence. Nevertheless the aim of placing children within their own extended family, or if not, with foster parents from the same community, is the same.

Community support programs should not discriminate between children whose parents died of AIDS and those whose parents died of other causes.

Mechanisms for the accountable distribution of small amounts of material support for households caring for orphans need to be established and the community encouraged to respond to the needs of orphans in a variety of ways.[9] It

9. R. S. Drew, C. Makufa, and G. Foster, "Strategies for Providing Care and Support to Children Orphaned by AIDS," *AIDS Care* 10 Suppl 1 (April 1998): S9–S15.

is important first to identify local community structures and leaders, such as women's groups, church groups, elected community representatives, and traditional leaders, and to understand how these structures relate to each other. Consultation with these groups and leaders can then help to identify a team who can be trained to train volunteers in mapping, enumeration, needs assessment, and support skills. Traditional and local political leadership may be invited to participate in the initial training sessions with the aim of enlisting their support. They may not train others but could help to create an environment in which all community members participate, drawing on traditional values and customs.

Those trained in the preliminary workshops could then facilitate community gatherings where selected volunteers work in local area groups to produce community maps and lists of households with orphans and children in need in their camp area or villages. They would discuss how to assess the needs of households with orphans or affected children, including the following:

- material needs: for shelter, food, clothes;
- emotional needs: for love, a sense of belonging, a sense of hope for the future, and comfort for bereavement;
- support needs: school fees, respite care, skills training, farming help;
- health care needs;
- recreational opportunities; and
- the need for protection against exploitation.[10]

An information system needs to be coordinated to collate and analyze trends in numbers of orphans and children in need and the size and types of households in which orphans live.

These needs might be met through volunteers undertaking to visit households regularly to provide support and through the establishment of day-care services that might provide recreation and meals. Respite baby care may enable older siblings to resume attending school, and volunteers with skills might be recruited to train young people. Microfinance programs can assist foster families. Collaboration with other sectors is vital and a long-term view is essential.

---

10. Convention on the Rights of the Child, 1990, *www.unicef .org.*

SUGGESTED INDICATORS

Indicator	*Method of measurement*
Home-based care	
Volunteers recruited and trained	Review of training records
Rate of turnover of home-based care volunteers	Review of register of volunteers
Proportion of PLWH who need home-based care receiving care	Door-to-door survey/local mapping with community members
Numbers of home-based care kits distributed	Review of records
Proportion of home-based carers aware of (1) availability of respite care and (2) referral procedures	Survey of home-based carers
Awareness of hospital doctors that home-based care is available	Review of discharge documents
Satisfaction of home-based care volunteers with level of support	In-depth interviews
Satisfaction of PLWH with home-based care system with PLWH receiving care at home	FGDs with PLWH; in-depth interviews
Clinic care	
Standard treatment protocols developed for common HIV-related conditions	Review of protocols
Proportion of PHC health care staff trained in management of HIV-related conditions	Review of training records
Proportion of health care staff who have received sensitization training, including the rights of PLWH	Review of training records
Hospital care	
Patients with HIV not segregated	Observation
Ethical hospital policies developed and disseminated	Review of policy documents Observation
Number of health professionals trained in diagnosis and management of HIV-related conditions	Review of records

SUGGESTED INDICATORS (CONTINUED)

Indicator	*Method of measurement*
Caring for carers	
Satisfaction of health care staff with support available	FGDs with staff; interviews with supervisors
Regular meetings held with health care staff	Recorded attendance at staff meetings
Orphan support	
Number of volunteers in each district/camp area trained in mapping, enumeration, and needs assessment	Review of records
Proportion of villages/areas with a register of orphan households	Review of registers
Number of home visits per month by volunteers	Review of volunteer logbooks
Number of orphan households provided with material assistance; type and quantity of material assistance provided	Review of accounts
Proportion of registered orphans malnourished (by gender); ratio of malnourished orphans to malnourished nonorphan children in specified age groups	Household survey
Proportion of orphans attending primary school	Household survey
Proportion of orphans participating in skills learning and recreational events	Household survey
Well-being of orphan households as assessed by members of the household including children	In-depth interviews

ADDITIONAL RESOURCES

Armstrong, S. *Caring for Carers: Managing Stress in Those Who Care for People with HIV and AIDS.* UNAIDS. *www.unaids.org.*

British National Formulary. Available at *www.bnf.org.* This is a very useful independent and reliable source of information about medicines.

Carpenter, C. J., et al. "Antiretroviral Therapy in Adults," *Journal of the American Medical Association* 283 (2000): 381.

Donahue, J., and J. Williamson. *Developing Interventions to Benefit Children and Families Affected by HIV/AIDS: A Review of the Cope Program in Malawi.* Washington, D.C.: USAID, Displaced Children and Orphans Fund, 1996.

France, N., et al. *Stigma, Denial, and Shame in Africa: Barriers to Community and Home-based Care for People Infected and Affected by HIV/AIDS.* First Regional Home- and Community-based Care Conference, Gaborone, Botswana, March 2001.

Holmes, W. *HIV Infection in Children (Sub-Saharan Africa).* 48-slide set with text. London: TALC, Institute of Child Health, 1992.

———. *HIV Infection — Clinical Manifestations in Adults (for the Asian and Pacific Region).* Slide set with text. London: TALC, Institute of Child Health, 1993.

Holmes, W., and F. Savage. *HIV Infection — Clinical Manifestations (for Sub-Saharan Africa).* Slide set with text. London: TALC, Institute of Child Health, 1988/89.

Hunter, S. *Building a Future for Families and Children Affected by HIV/AIDS: Report on a Two-year Project for Care and Protection Programs for Children Affected by HIV/AIDS.* New York: UNICEF/Child Protection Division, 1999.

Hunter, S., and J. Williamson. *Children on the Brink: Strategies to Support Children Isolated by HIV/AIDS.* Washington, D.C.: USAID, 1997.

Mariasy, Judith. *Triple Jeopardy: Women and AIDS.* London: Panos Publications, 1990.

Miller, D. *Key Elements in HIV/AIDS Care and Support.* WHO/UNAIDS, September 2000. *www.unaids.org.*

Stewart, G., ed. *Could It Be HIV? The Clinical Recognition of HIV Infection.* Kingsgrove, NSW: Australasian Medical Publishing Company, 1993.

Strategies for Hope Series. *The Orphan Generation.* Video about community-based care and support for orphans in Uganda. Available from TALC.

———. *Under the Mapundu Tree.* A video about a home care program in Zambia. Available from TALC. *www.stratshope.org.*

UNAIDS. "AIDS: Palliative Care." October 2000. *www.unaids.org.*

———. *Comfort and Hope: Six Case Studies on Mobilizing Family and Community Care for and by People with HIV/AIDS.* June 1999.

———. *Developing HIV/AIDS Treatment Guidelines.* Geneva, 1999.

———. "Provisional WHO/UNAIDS Secretariat Recommendations on the Use of Co-trimoxazole Prophylaxis in Adults and Children Living with HIV/AIDS in Africa." September 2000. *www.unaids.org.*

———. "Sources and Prices of Selected Drugs and Diagnostics for People Living with HIV/AIDS." May 2001. *www.supply.unicef.dk.*

UNAIDS/WHO. "Tuberculosis and AIDS: UNAIDS Best Practice Collection." WHO Policy Statement on Preventive Therapy against Tuberculosis in PLWH.

UNICEF. *Principles to Guide Programming for Orphans and Other Vulnerable Children.* New York: UNICEF, 2001.

USAID. *Community Mobilization to Mitigate the Impacts of HIV/AIDS.* Washington, D.C.: USAID Displaced Children and Orphans Fund, 1999.

WHO. *Scaling Up Antiretroviral Therapy in Resource Limited Settings: Guidelines for a Public Health Approach.* Geneva: WHO, 2002.

———. *Tuberculosis Control in Refugee Situations: An Inter-Agency Field Manual.* Geneva: WHO/TB/97. 221, 1997.

WHO/GPA. *AIDS Home Care Handbook.* WHO/GPA/IDS/HCS/93.2, 1993.

———. "Guidelines for the Clinical Management of HIV Infection in Adults." *Gpa/ids/hcs/91.6,* 1991.

———. "Guidelines for the Clinical Management of HIV Infection in Children." *Gpa/ids/hcs/93.3,* November 1993.

Appendix A

Questions to Assist in Planning a Situation Analysis

These are general questions from which you can prepare questions for a questionnaire survey or question guides for focus group discussions. It is important for the situation analysis team to think about the topics and questions that will be most relevant and appropriate in their particular setting.

Demographic and socioeconomic data

- How large is the displaced population? the host population?

- Over what geographic area is the population distributed?

- What is the composition of the population in terms of age, sex, ethnic, language, religious, educational, and socioeconomic characteristics?

- What are the characteristics of the local population?

- What is the range of household structures and the average household size?

- What are the sources and levels of income? Is there much inequality in household income and living standards?

- What is the level of mobility into and out of the population, and what are the reasons for these movements?

Local decision-making structures and processes, gender relations, networks, interest groups, and elites

- How is the refugee/IDP population living? in camps, with host families, in informal settlements?

This appendix is adapted from T. Aboagye-Kwarteng, R. Moodie, and W. Holme, *Community Action on HIV: A Resource Manual for Prevention, Care and Support,* 2d ed. (Melbourne: Macfarlane Burnet Institute for Medical Research and Public Health, 2000).

- How is the displaced population organized and what is their status? Who has responsibility for supplies, services, and protecting their rights?

- Who has power in this population and how do they exercise it? Who are the formal and informal leaders of the community? How are they appointed or chosen? What role do religious groups and traditional structures play? What are relationships like between the various community structures?

- Are there military groups present? What are the relationships between different military groups?

- Does the refugee/IDP population have access to land and employment and to services such as education, health, and transport? Are some groups within the refugee/IDP population marginalized?

- How do the roles, status, and power of men and women differ? How have they changed as a result of displacement? How do cultural expectations of men's and women's roles affect the lives of men and women?

- How common is domestic violence? (A useful question is to ask whether the respondent has been hit by someone in his or her home in the past month.)

- How much mixing is there between the refugee/IDP and the local population, and what form does this take?

- How and where do people gather to talk about issues of importance to the community?

- What is the influence of the seasons on the lives of the refugees/IDPs?

Opportunities for communication

- Where do refugees or the displaced population obtain their information? through newspapers, radio, word-of-mouth?

- What sources of information do people trust?

- What methods of communicating information are available?

- What proportion of the population can read (by age and gender)?

- Are there different language groups among the refugees/IDPs?

- How many people own or can listen to a radio? Who listens to the radio, how often, and at what times of day? What programs do people of different ages and gender prefer? What different types of radio stations are there?

The health status of the community

- What are the main causes of death? Are there any estimates on how this varies according to age, gender, and setting?

- What are the main causes of illness (by age, gender, and setting)?

- What are the levels of disability in the community?

Distribution and frequency of HIV infection and other sexually transmitted infections

- What types of STIs are common? Enquire about ulcerative STIs such as syphilis, chancroid, herpes, and granuloma inguinale, and STIs that cause discharge such as gonorrhea and chlamydia.

- How are STIs treated and reported? Is laboratory diagnosis available or are health care workers trained in syndromic management of STIs? Is there any system for contact tracing? Is HIV testing provided? Is it confidential? Is pre- and post-test counseling available?

- What are the incidence and the prevalence of STIs, and what are the trends? (Incidence is the number of new cases in the population over a given period of time, and prevalence is the number of cases in the population at any given time.)

- Is there any survey or sentinel surveillance data about prevalence of HIV?

Access to and use of health care and welfare services

- What types of health services are provided for women, men, and children?

- Who provides the services — government, religious or secular NGOs, private doctors, pharmacies, traditional healers, street vendors?

- Who is using health services? Are there any statistics available, by age, sex, location, type of service? How accessible, acceptable, and affordable are these services? What are the barriers to their use?

- What are the most important cultural beliefs, including religious, social, family, and political beliefs, that influence health behaviors?

- What support is available for single pregnant women?

- How are orphans and children without families cared for?

Young people[1]

- What are the cultural norms related to sexual relationships and rites of passage into adulthood (including harmful traditional practices, such as female genital mutilation)?

- What are the typical patterns of adult authority over adolescents?

- What services are there for young people? What are the barriers to their access?

- What are the perceptions of camp staff and service providers related to providing health services to young people?

- How do young people perceive their reproductive health needs?

---

1. See *Reproductive Health in Refugee Situations: Inter-Agency Field Manual*, 1999.

Care and support for people with HIV infection

- What health and support services are available for people with chronic illness?

- Are any counseling services available? What are the training needs for counselors?

- What are the traditional patterns of care for people with chronic illness?

- How open is the community about HIV? Are there PLWH who are open about their status? How are they treated?

- What are the most urgent needs of PLWH?

- What treatments are available for HIV-related symptoms and for opportunistic infections? Is any kind of palliative care available for the dying?

- Do people have to pay for health care, including medicines?

- Where are people with HIV-related disease being cared for? How far do they have to travel, and at what cost?

- Are there any support groups for people living with HIV infection or AIDS?

- Are PLWH involved in planning and implementing HIV prevention and care activities?

- Is support available for family members, volunteers, and health care workers who care for people with HIV-related illness?

Patterns of sexual behavior

- What are the traditional societal and cultural attitudes and rules about sex? How do these differ for men and for women? Is there a difference between attitudes toward sexual behavior expressed publicly and what people do in private?

- What social opportunities are available for the displaced population that enable people of opposite sexes to meet?

- Has the gender and age structure of the displaced population changed significantly, leaving an excess of single men or single women? What impact is this having on patterns of sexual behavior?

- At what age do young people start to have sex and what are their patterns of sexual behavior — has this changed as a result of being displaced?

- Who do young people learn about sex from?

- How common is transactional sex, that is, when sex is exchanged for money, goods, or protection?

- How is sex work organized? Who controls sex work? Do sex workers have access to health care services and to condoms? Do they have their own organizations?

- How common is coerced sex?

- How common is sexual violence and sexual abuse? for women? for men? for young women, for young men? for children? When and where does it occur? How can the vulnerable be protected against sexual violence?

- What support is available for refugees/IDPs who have been raped or sexually assaulted?

- What are the common attitudes toward homosexuality? Where and when do men have sex with men?

- Is there sexual contact between the displaced and the local populations, between the military and the displaced population?

- What is the level of knowledge about STIs and HIV? What are the common misconceptions?

- What is the level of concern and beliefs about the consequences of sex — STIs, infertility, and unwanted pregnancies?

- What is the level of knowledge, use of, and access to contraception and family planning?

- What are the major influences on sexual behavior and attitudes for men, women, and young people?

- How common are sexual activities that increase risk? These include anal sex, dry sex, beating or traumatic sex, sex during menstruation, and sex during pregnancy.

- How common are sexual activities that decrease risk? These include nonpenetrative sex, such as sex between the thighs, massage, mutual masturbation, and oral sex.

- What are knowledge, attitudes, and practice in relation to condoms? What are the availability, cost, accessibility, and quality of condoms? Can women access condoms? Can young unmarried people access condoms? Are female condoms available and acceptable?

- Do couples have sex during pregnancy? After childbirth?

- Has concern about HIV influenced sexual behavior and practices? Management of blood safety and infection control?

- How frequent are blood transfusions, who gives them, and for what reasons? Are criteria to minimize the use of transfusions established?

- Is there a blood bank system in operation?

- Are blood donors volunteers, paid, or family members of the patient?

- Is blood for transfusion screened for antibodies to HIV, hepatitis, and syphilis?

- What are the training needs in relation to blood safety?

- Are appropriate universal infection control practices followed in health care settings?

- What are the training needs of health care workers and traditional healers and birth attendants in relation to infection control?

Exploring risk
from injecting drug use

- Is injecting drug use known to occur among the displaced population? Was it a problem in the country of origin? Is it a problem among the local population?

- Are drugs grown or produced in the area, e.g., opium poppies or amphetamines? Are injectable drugs transported through the area?

- What is the estimated number of people who inject drugs? Is this increasing?

- Do people take drugs by other routes — such as smoking or by mouth?

- Who injects drugs, and in what circumstances? What are their reasons?

- Are there estimates of HIV infection and other blood-borne viruses, hepatitis B, and hepatitis C, among those who inject?

- Are the sexual partners of people who inject becoming infected with HIV and other blood-borne viruses?

- What are the common attitudes toward those who inject drugs? Are they stigmatized and rejected?

- Is there a strong link between injecting drug use and commercial sex work?

- How do people inject? With what equipment? How many people do they share with? Where do they do it?

- Do injecting drug users make efforts to avoid HIV, for example, by not sharing, by rinsing needles and syringes, by boiling needles and syringes, or by using bleach to clean their needles and syringes? Is bleach available?

- How easy is it to get needles and syringes?

- Are there any treatment or rehabilitation services available for those addicted to drugs? If so, what type of services are they, and where are they situated?

- What are the attitudes of the police toward those who inject?

Knowledge, beliefs, and practice
in relation to pregnancy, childbirth,
and infant feeding

- What are the cultural beliefs in relation to pregnancy, childbirth, the post-partum period, and infant feeding? How have these been affected by the displacement?

- Who makes decisions in relation to pregnancy, attendance at prenatal care, delivery care, and infant feeding? Is it the woman, her husband, her mother-in-law, or other family members?

- What are the likely consequences if a pregnant woman discloses a positive HIV test result to her family?

- What are the influences on breast-feeding practices? How common is exclusive breast-feeding?

- Are there any practical, safe, affordable, and acceptable alternatives to breast-feeding in this setting?

- What were weaning food practices before the emergency, and what are the current infant feeding practices?

- How are sick babies cared for?

Laws that relate to HIV and other STIs

- What laws are the refugee/IDP population subject to that relate to prevention and care of HIV? How are these laws interpreted and enforced?

- Are there legal requirements to notify government officials about individuals with HIV infection or AIDS? Are they reported with their full name and address or with a code? Is it a confidential system?

- Is mandatory testing for HIV antibodies forbidden?

- Is disclosure of information about people with HIV or STIs forbidden? Is there a law that requires individuals infected with HIV to tell their sexual partner that they have HIV?

- Are there laws against discrimination on the basis of health status (including HIV infection), gender, sexual preference, political views, and religion?

- Do women have the legal right to inherit or own property, particularly after the death of a spouse?

- Are there broadcasting, censorship, or obscenity laws that prevent the dissemination of frank messages about HIV, STIs, and sexual and drug injecting behavior?

- How is rape defined in law, and what are the penalties?

- Is termination of pregnancy legal? Under what circumstances?

- Is prostitution illegal? Are there laws against living on the earnings of prostitution or running a brothel?

- Is homosexuality an offense? Is this law enforced?

- What are the laws relating to production, trafficking, and possession of drugs, and to equipment used for injecting, such as needles and syringes, swabs, and spoons?

Appendix B

HIV Testing Strategies

The use of a combination of rapid and simple tests can avoid the use of expensive tests such as the Western blot for confirmation. WHO and UNAIDS have recommended HIV testing strategies according to test objective and prevalence of infection in the population (see the table at the foot of this page).

STRATEGY ONE

A sample which tests positive can be counted as positive for the purpose of surveillance, or rejected as positive for the purpose of screening for transfusion. However, if the donor is to be informed of the result then proceed as for "Identification of asymptomatic HIV-infected people" with strategy two or three depending on the prevalence of HIV.

If the sample tests negative, then the result can be reported as negative to the donor (with post-test counseling).

STRATEGY TWO

If the sample tests negative, then the result can be reported as negative to the client/patient (with post-test counseling).

If the sample tests positive on the first test, repeat the test with a different type of test based on a different antigen preparation or different testing principle.

If the second test is also positive the result can be reported to the client/patient, with counseling.

For samples which have tested positive on the first test and negative on the second test:

- Retest the sample with the same two tests.

- If both tests are positive the second time, confirm that a second sample is positive. Then tell the client/patient that the test result is positive and proceed with counseling.

- If both tests are negative the second time, tell the persons that they have a negative test result and counsel them.

HIV TESTING STRATEGIES

Reason for HIV antibody test	HIV prevalence	Testing Strategy
Identification of asymptomatic HIV-infected people	< 10% > 10%	3 2
Diagnosis of HIV-related disease	< 30% > 30%	3 2
Epidemiological surveillance	< 10% > 10%	2 1
Screening blood for transfusion	All prevalences	1

—"UNAIDS and WHO Recommendations for HIV Testing Strategies," *Weekly Epidemiological Record,* no. 12, March 21, 1997.

- If the two test results still differ then consider the result uncertain or "indeterminate." Repeat this testing strategy on a different sample taken fourteen days later.

STRATEGY THREE

If the sample tests negative, then the result can be reported as negative to the client/patient, with counseling.

If the sample tests positive on the first test repeat the test with a different type of test based on a different antigen preparation or different testing principle.

If the second test is also positive the result can be reported to the client/patient, with counseling.

For samples which have tested positive on the first test and negative on the second test:

- Retest the sample with the same two tests.

- If both tests are positive the second time, then test the sample with a third different test.

- If the third test gives a positive result, confirm that a second sample is positive. Then tell the client/patient that they have a positive test result and counsel them.

- If the third test is negative then consider the result uncertain or "indeterminate." Repeat this testing strategy on a different sample taken fourteen days later.

- If one test is positive and one test is negative, then test the sample with a third different test.

- If the third test gives a positive result, then consider the result uncertain or "indeterminate." Repeat this testing strategy on a different sample taken fourteen days later.

- If the third test gives a negative result and the client/patient has been at risk of HIV infection in the previous three months, then consider the result uncertain or "indeterminate." Repeat this testing strategy on a different sample taken fourteen days later.

- If the third test gives a negative result and the client/patient has not been at risk of HIV infection in the previous three months, tell the client/patient that they have a negative test result and counsel them (but do not use their blood for transfusion).

Appendix C

PLA Exercises for Gathering Sensitive Information — Some Examples

WHAT QUALITIES DO WE LIKE IN THE OPPOSITE SEX — AND WHY?

This exercise is designed to generate discussion about gender roles and relations and increase understanding about the choices that young people make.

Identify someone in the team who is good at drawing. You can use or adapt the pictures on the following two pages as a guide to make two sets of picture cards that illustrate a range of characteristics for each sex. For example:

Boys	*Girls*
Good-looking	Pretty
Brave	Brave
Cheeky	Sexy
Bold	Shy
Arrogant	Vain
Clever	Clever
Jealous	Jealous
Responsible	Responsible
Kind	Kind
Rich	Rich
Poor	Poor
Respectful	Respectful
Aggressive	Quarrelsome
Generous	Good cook
Angry	Angry
Strong	Smart (fashionable)
Likes children	Likes children
Affectionate/Caring	Caring/affectionate
Funny	Funny
Popular	Popular
Sporty	Modern
Smart (fashionable)	Sporty
Funny	Funny
Daring	Daring

You can use these cards in a number of participatory exercises.

You might ask the boys and girls to get into separate sex groups. Ask each group to rank the cards in answer to the following questions:

- What characteristics does a boy look for in a girlfriend? and why?
- What characteristics does a girl look for in a boyfriend? and why?
- What characteristics does a boy look for in a potential wife? and why?
- What characteristics does a girl look for in a potential husband? and why?

After each "round" you could encourage each group to "visit" the work of the other group. This will generate a lot of discussion and increase understanding of how boys and girls view each other.

This is a useful exercise to have before a discussion or information-gathering exercise about sexual behavior.

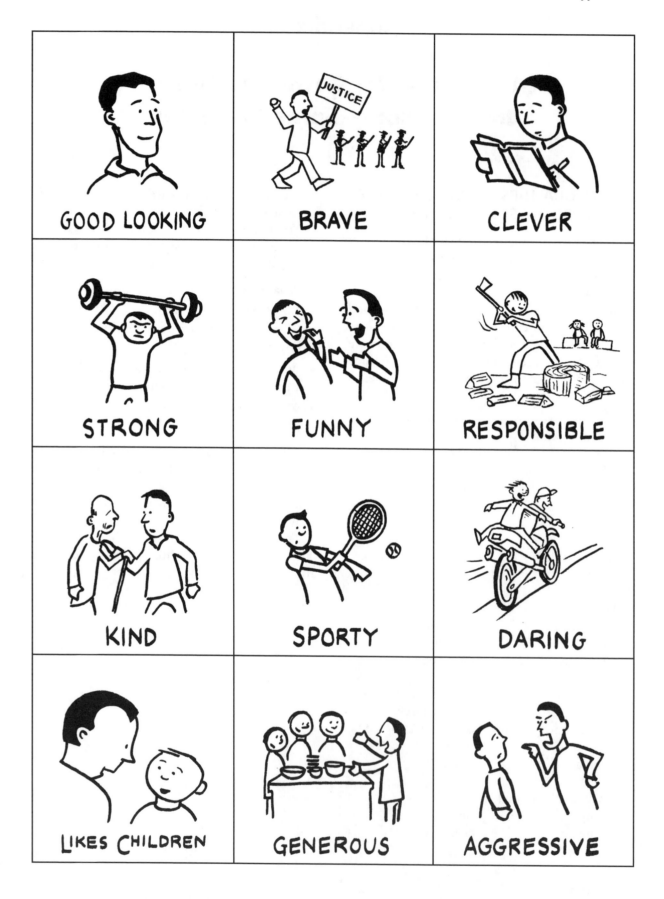

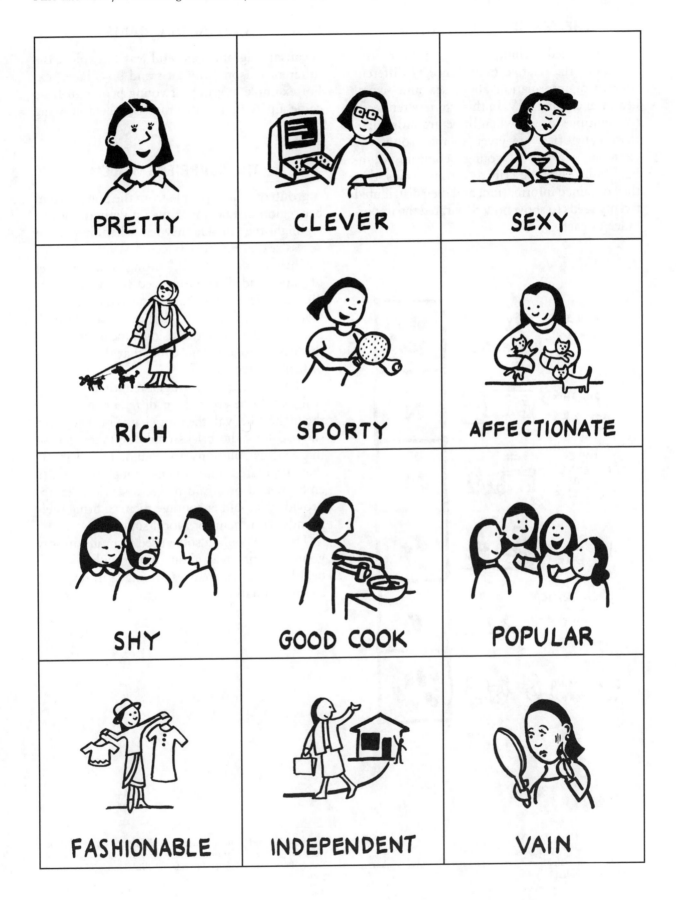

THE TEN SEED TECHNIQUE

The "ten seed technique" is useful for asking about the relative importance of different sources of information about sex and sexual health, including HIV. In this exercise ten seeds (or multiples of ten when there are more than three categories) are given to the group. For example, a group of young people in Mumbai, India, first described various ways that they obtained information, and then distributed twenty seeds to show how they rated the importance of each.[1]

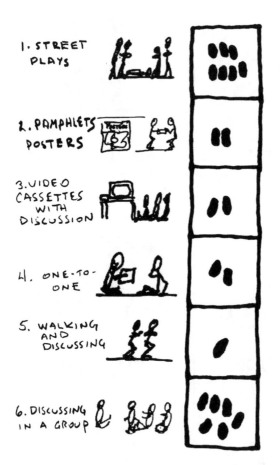

1. STREET PLAYS

2. PAMPHLETS POSTERS

3. VIDEO CASSETTES WITH DISCUSSION

4. ONE-TO-ONE

5. WALKING AND DISCUSSING

6. DISCUSSING IN A GROUP

CAUSAL DIAGRAMS

A causal diagram is a useful way to explore the different reasons why girls and boys have sex. For example, a group of young people in Laos came up with the diagram on the following page.

THE "BARRIERS WALL"

A group of young people from the South Humber region of England came up with an idea to highlight the barriers they feel when they try to access sexual health services.[2]

They made a "wall," using a large sheet of paper and differently sized sticky cards for "bricks." The cards could be moved or replaced several times during the discussion. Each brick represented a barrier to using a local service, in this case a government clinic that they felt was difficult to access.

The young people suggested that separate walls could be created for different services — the higher the wall the more barriers. They also showed how the bricks could be taken out of the wall as solutions are found. For example they suggested that when young people are embarrassed or afraid to use a service, service providers should encourage them to bring their friends with them for moral support.

This tool could also be used to monitor how young people feel about a particular sexual health service as changes are made in response to the evaluation.

---

1. From an evaluation exercise conducted by Ravi Jayakaran, World Vision India.

2. M. Westerby and T. Sellers, "Evaluating Sexual Health Services in the UK: Adapting Participatory Appraisal Tools with Young People and Service Providers," *PLA Notes* 37 (February 2000).

REASONS FOR HAVING SEX

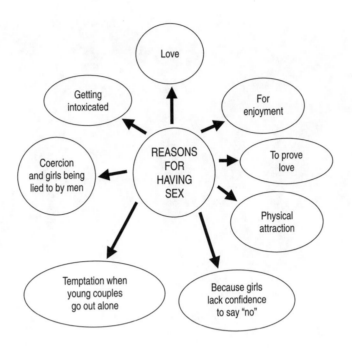

BARRIERS WALL

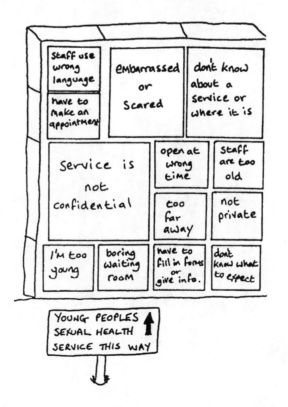

Appendix D

Syndromic Management of Sexually Transmitted Infections

Both men and women can have gonorrhea or chlamydia without any signs. Gonorrhea and chlamydia can have the same signs, though gonorrhea usually starts sooner and is more painful.

Cervicitis means inflammation of the cervix of the uterus. It can be caused by gonorrhea or chlamydia. A woman can have gonorrhea and chlamydia at the same time so it is best to treat for both.

In a man the signs of urethral discharge can begin as early as two to five days after he has sex with an infected person. But in a woman the signs may not begin for weeks or even months.

Signs

- yellow or green discharge from the vagina, penis, or anus,
- pain or burning during urination,
- pain in the lower abdomen,
- fever,
- pain during sex.

Management

See the flow chart on page 208 for syndromic management of vaginal and urethral discharge.

SORES (ULCERS) ON THE GENITALS (SYPHILIS, CHANCROID, HERPES)

Most sores or ulcers on the genitals are caused by having sex with an infected person. A single painless sore is a sign of syphilis. But if there is more than one sore, and they are painful, it is likely to be another STI such as chancroid or genital herpes. It is important to keep any genital sores clean until they are healed and to avoid sex.

See online *www.who.int/docstore/hiv/STIManagemntguidelines/ who_hiv_aids_2001.01/* for WHO's "Guidelines for the Management of Sexually Transmitted Infections."

Syphilis

Syphilis is a common and dangerous disease. A pregnant woman with syphilis can pass the infection to her unborn child.

Signs

The first sign is a sore called a chancre. It appears two to five weeks after sexual contact with a person with syphilis. The chancre may look like a pimple, a blister, or an open sore. It usually appears on the genital area of a man or a woman, but it might appear on the lips, fingers, anus, or mouth. This sore is full of organisms which are easily passed on to another person. The sore is usually painless, and if it is inside the vagina a woman may not know that she has it, but she can still infect others.

The sore lasts only for a few days or weeks. It then goes away by itself without treatment. But the disease continues spreading through the body.

Weeks or months later there may be a sore throat, mild fever, mouth sores, swollen joints, or skin rashes. During this stage the disease can be spread by simple physical contact, such as kissing or touching, because the organisms are on the skin.

All of the above signs usually go away by themselves, and then the individuals often think they are well. But the disease continues. Without proper treatment syphilis can invade any part of the body causing heart disease, paralysis, insanity, and sometimes death.

Management

See the flow chart on page 213 for syndromic management of genital ulcers.

207

FLOW CHART FOR VAGINAL DISCHARGE SYNDROME

Patient complains of vaginal discharge

Risk assessment:

- Complaint of lower abdominal pain or
- Partner has symptoms or
- Risk factor positive

NO

- Treat for vaginitis
- Educate for behavior change
- Offer HIV counseling and testing if facilities available
- Promote/provide condoms

YES

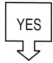

- Treat for cervicitis (gonorrhea and chlamydia) and vaginitis
- Educate for behavior change
- Promote/provide condoms
- Partner management
- Advise to return if necessary

Chancroid

These sores appear three to five days after sexual relations with an infected person. Each sore begins as a soft, painful pimple, which quickly opens up to become a shallow ulcer with ragged edges. The ulcer is usually red around the outside edges.

Signs

- soft painful sores on the genitals or anus;
- enlarged lymph nodes in the groin.

Management

See the flow chart for syndromic management of genital ulcers below. Remember to suggest that the woman's partner be treated at the same time. Enlarged nodes in the groin may need to be incised.

Genital herpes

Genital herpes is a painful skin infection caused by a virus and spread from person to person during sex. Small blisters appear on the genitals and sometimes on the mouth. You can also get herpes sores on the mouth that are not spread by sex (cold sores).

Signs

- A tingling, itching, or painful feeling of the skin is present in the genital area or thighs.

EXAMPLES OF TREATMENT OPTIONS FOR VAGINAL DISCHARGE SYNDROME

Treatment for vaginitis:

Metronidazole 500 mg, twice daily for 7 days

Treatment for cervicitis:

Gonorrhea

ciprofloxacin* 500 mg orally, as a single oral dose

or

azithromycin 1 g orally, as a single dose

or

ceftriaxone, 125 mg im, as a single dose

or

cefixime, 400 mg orally, as a single dose

or

spectinomycin, 2 g im, as a single dose

Alternatives:

kanamycin. 2 g im, as a single dose

or

cotrimoxazole 80/400 mg, 10 tablets orally, once a day for 3 days

---

Chlamydia

azithromycin 1 g single dose

or

doxycycline* 100 mg, twice daily for 10 days

or

erythromycin 500 mgs orally 4 times daily for 7 days

Alternatives:

amoxycillin, 500 mg orally, 3 times a day for 7 days

or

ofloxacin, 300 mg orally, twice daily for 7 days

or

tetracycline*, 500 mg orally, 4 times a day for 7 days

---

*contraindicated in pregnancy

- One or more small, very painful blisters appear on the genitals, anus, buttocks, or thighs.

- The blisters bursts and form small, red open sores that are very painful.

- The sores dry up and become scabs.

The first time someone gets herpes sores it can last for two weeks or more — with fever, headache, body ache, chills, and swollen lymph nodes in the groin. There may be pain on urination.

The virus stays in the body after all the signs have gone away. New blisters can appear at any time, from weeks to years later. Usually the new sores appear in the same place. But there are not as many, they are less painful, and they usually heal faster.

People with AIDS can get herpes anywhere on their body, and it may take longer to get better.

Management

There is no cure for herpes. But there are some things a person can do to feel better.

Pour cool clean water over the genitals when passing urine. This helps to stop the burning. Soak some cloths in cool black tea and put them on the sore. Sit in a pan or bath of clean, cool water. Give paracetamol 500 mgs every four hours for pain or aspirin 600 mgs four hourly.

Advise the woman to wash her hands frequently and not touch her eyes because the infection can spread to the eyes.

A pregnant woman with herpes sores can pass the virus to the baby during childbirth. The virus is very dangerous to the baby. It is best for women with herpes to have a caesarean section.

FLOW CHART FOR VAGINAL DISCHARGE
WITH SPECULUM

Patient complains of vaginal discharge

Risk assessment:

- Complaint of lower abdominal pain or
- Partner has symptoms or
- Risk factor positive?

No → Speculum available? → **No** →

- Treat for vaginitis
- Educate for behavior change
- Offer HIV counseling and testing if facilities available
- Promote/provide condoms

Yes ↓

- Treat for chlamydia, gonorrhea, and vaginitis
- Educate for behavior change
- Offer HIV counseling and testing if facilities available
- Promote/provide condoms
- Partner management
- Advise to return if necessary

Yes ↓

Mucopus from cervix? → Treat for gonorrhea and chlamydia (cervicitis)

Profuse discharge? → Treat for trichomonas

Curd-like discharge? → Treat for candida

EXAMPLES OF TREATMENT OPTIONS FOR
TRICHOMONAS VAGINALIS AND *CANDIDA ALBICANS*

Treatment for *Trichomonas vaginalis* vaginal infection:

metronidazole, 2 g orally, as a single dose
    or
tinidazole, 2 g orally, as a single dose

Alternatives:
metronidazole, 400 or 500 mg orally, twice daily for 7 days
    or
tinidazole, 500 mg orally, twice daily for 5 days.

Note: patients taking the above drugs should be cautioned not to consume alcohol during the treatment and for 24 hours after the last dose.

Treatment for *Candida albicans*:

miconazole or clotrimazole, 200 mg intravaginally, daily for 3 days
    or
clotrimazole, 500 mg intravaginally, as a single dose
    or
fluconazole, 150 mg orally, as a single dose

Alternative:
nystatin, 100,000 IU intravaginally, daily for 14 days

FLOW CHART FOR URETHRAL DISCHARGE SYNDROME

Patient complains of urethral discharge

Take history and examine
Milk urethra if necessary

Discharge confirmed

 No

- Educate for behavior change
- Offer HIV counseling and testing if facilities available
- Promote/provide condoms

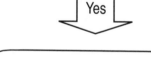 Yes

- Treat for chlamydia and gonorrhea
- Educate for behavior change
- Offer HIV counseling and testing if facilities available
- Promote/provide condoms
- Partner management
- Advise to return in seven days

FLOW CHART FOR GENITAL ULCER SYNDROME

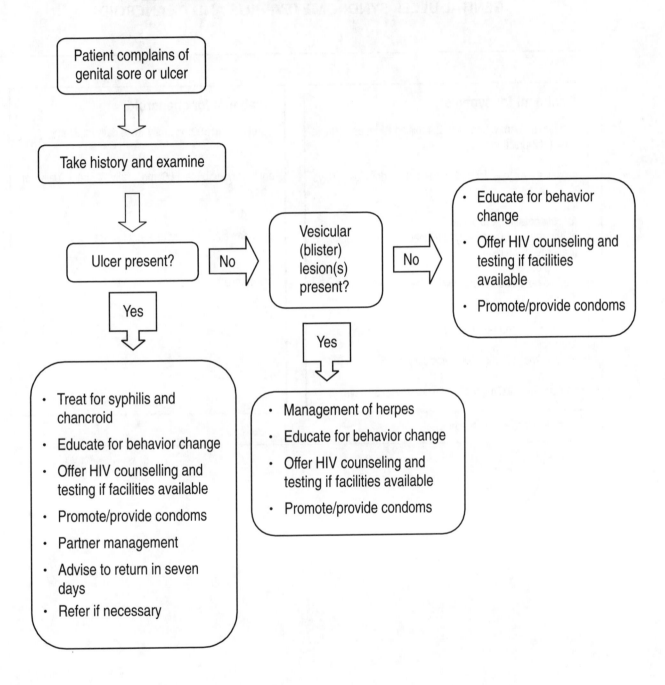

EXAMPLES OF TREATMENT OPTIONS FOR
GENITAL ULCER SYNDROME (SYPHILIS AND CHANCROID)

Treatment for syphilis

benzathine benzyl penicillin, 2.4 million IU im as a single dose (at 2 injection sites)
            or
procaine benzylpenicillin, 1.2 million IU im daily for 10 days
            or

for patients allergic to penicillin
erythromycin 500 mg orally four times a day for 15 days (if allergy to penicillin)
            plus
cotrimoxazole 80/400 mg, two tablets orally, twice daily for 7 days

Alternative for non-pregnant patients who are allergic to penicillin:
doxycycline* 100 mg orally twice daily for 15 days
            or
tetracycline*, 500 mg orally, 4 times daily for 30 days

*contraindicated in pregnancy

Treatment for chancroid:

ciprofloxacin* 500 mg orally, twice daily for 3 days

        or

erythromycin base 500 mg orally, 4 times daily for 7 days

        or

azithromycin, 1 g orally, as a single dose

Alternative:

ceftriaxone, 250 mg im, as a single dose

Appendix E

Selected References, Resources, and Further Reading

MANUALS AND GUIDELINES

Clinical Tuberculosis, by John Crofton, Norman Horne, and Fred Miller. Available from TALC (address on page 217).

Community Action on HIV: A Resource Manual for Prevention, Care, and Support. Melbourne: Macfarlane Burnet Institute for Medical Research and Public Health, 2001 (*community@burnet.edu.au*).

Expanding the Global Response to HIV/AIDS through Focused Action Reducing Risk and Vulnerability: Definitions, Rationale, and Pathways. UNAIDS.

Facilitating Sustainable Behaviour Change. Bruce Parnell and Kim Benton. A guidebook for designing HIV programs. Melbourne: Macfarlane Burnet Institute for Medical Research and Public Health, 1999 (*community@burnet.edu.au*).

Fact Sheets on HIV/AIDS for nurses and midwives. WHO. *www.who.int.*

Guidelines for HIV Interventions in Emergency Settings. UNAIDS, 1998. *www.unaids.org.*

Mental Health of Refugees. Geneva, WHO, and the UNHCR, 134 pp. This manual focuses on specific learning objectives for relief workers. It gives practical advice on how to help refugees and displaced people through counseling, self-help groups, modern drugs, and traditional medicine. A special section on refugee children is included.

Migrant Populations and HIV/AIDS: The Development and Implementation of Programmes: Theory, Methodology and Practice. Geneva: UNAIDS, 2000. *www.unaids.org.* HIV Prevention and AIDS in Africa. Royal Tropical Institute (KIT). Amsterdam: Royal Tropical Institute (KIT): 1997. US$ 25.00 from Mr. Max Mink. *kitpress@mail.support.nl.*

Preventing a Crisis, by Gill Gordon and Tony Klouda. Available from TALC (address on page 217).

Refugee Health: An Approach to Emergency Situations. Médecins Sans Frontières. London: Macmillan/ TALC/Médecins Sans Frontières; 1997. An invaluable guide to many aspects of refugee/IDP health. Has a brief chapter on STIs and HIV.

Refugee Reproductive Health. Reproductive Health Outlook. Program for Appropriate Technology in Health. *www.rho.org.* Provides a useful overview with links to useful publications.

Reproductive Health Issues in Refugee Settings. Care International, Atlanta, Georgia, 1996. This five-day training module for health personnel focuses on skills learning and includes information on family planning, HIV/AIDS/STI, sexual and gender violence, maternal care, safe motherhood, and obstetric emergencies.

Reproductive Health in Refugee Situations: Inter-Agency Field Manual. Reproductive Health for Refugees Consortium website at *www.rhrc.org* lists Field Tools available on the site including this Inter-Agency Field Manual. Other field tools available on the site are:

- Training
- Needs Assessment Field Tools
- Reproductive Health During Conflict and Displacement, WHO
- UNFPA Reproductive Health Kit for Emergency Situations: Information on ordering the supplies and equipment
- Sexual Violence in Refugee Crises: a synopsis of the UNHCR Guidelines for prevention and response

"The Reproductive Health of Refugees: Special Supplement," ed. Laurel Shreck, *International Family Planning Perspectives* 26 (2000): 161–92.

Resource Package for HIV/AIDS in Refugee Situations. Geneva: UNHCR, January 1999. This resource pack contains: the UNHCR policy statement on HIV/AIDS in refugee/IDP situations; the UNHCR/UNAIDS Cooperation Framework; an HIV/AIDS programming checklist; the UNAIDS document request form; UNAIDS, Technical Updates and Points of View; Guidelines on HIV/AIDS Interventions in Refugee Settings; and an HIV/AIDS epidemic up-date. *www.unhcr.ch.*

Second Generation Surveillance for HIV. Compilation of Basic Materials. On CD ROM. UNAIDS/WHO Working group on Global HIV/AIDS and STI Surveillance. January 2001. WHO/CDS/CSR/EDC/2000.8. Available from WHO/UNAIDS.

Sexual Health and Health Care: Care and Support for People With HIV/AIDS in Resource-Poor Settings, Health and Population Occasional Paper, 1998. C. Gilks. A 192-page guidance book for planners and policy makers on how best to utilize scarce financial and human resources for health and disease, specifically HIV/AIDS care and prevention, promoting positive attitudes for care and support for people living with HIV/AIDS; examples from developing countries are provided. DFID fax 44-20-7336-6688 (*info@ifh.org.uk*).

Sexual Violence against Refugees: Guidelines on Prevention and Response. Geneva: UNHCR, 1995, 99pp. (English and French). This booklet describes when and how sexual violence can occur in the refugee/IDP context, its effects, and basic practical advice in areas of medical treatment, psychological support, and legal intervention.

Stepping Stones: A Training Package on HIV/AIDS, Communication and Relationship Skills. Alice Welbourn. Strategies for Hope, London: ActionAid, 1995 (*mail@actionaid.org.uk*). Available from TALC (address on page 217).

Surveillance in Emergency Situations. Brussels: Médecins Sans Frontières, 1993, 46pp. This practical guide describes how to set up a surveillance system in the early stages of an emergency situation, especially in refugee or displaced person camps.

UNAIDS best practice reports *www.unaids.org.*

Women and AIDS. An international resource book by Marge Berer with Sunanda Ray Available from TALC (address on page 217).

NEWSLETTERS

AIDS Action. Published four times a year.

Child Health Dialogue. Published four times a year; concentrates on international pediatric health promotion and disease prevention in relation to acute respiratory infections, diarrhea, malaria, malnutrition, and measles.

Health Action. Published three times a year, emphasizes international implementation of primary health care.

These excellent newsletters, all published by **Healthlink Worldwide,** include practical information, case studies, and training ideas and provide a forum for questions and exchange of ideas. They are available as hard copies by subscription, in PDF format at *www.healthlink.org.uk,* or by e-mail text (recent editions only).

Single copies of most of Healthlink Worldwide's publications are FREE to individuals and indigenous organizations in developing countries. For others, payment is required with order. See postal address below. E-mail: *publications@healthlink.org.uk.*

How to get e-mail text versions of the newsletters: The text without illustrations is available by e-mail from HealthNet, a communications network administered by SatelLife linking health workers in developing countries and other parts of the world. This service is particularly useful in situations where it is hard to receive attachments or download documents from the web. To subscribe to the e-mail text version of AIDS Action write to: *robin@usa.healthnet.org* and in the body of your message, type: "subscribe aids-action" for AIDS Action; "subscribe

chd" for Child Health Dialogue; "subscribe health action" for Health Action.

—

Very useful, comprehensive, and well-referenced population reports are available on the Internet or free of charge (single or multiple copies) from **John Hopkins University, Population Reports,** 111 Market Place, Suite 310, Baltimore, MD 21202-4024, USA.

Examples:

Closing the Condom Gap (vol. 27, no. 1, April 1999), series H, no. 9.

GATHER Guide to Counseling (vol. 26, no. 4, December 1998), series J, no. 48.

Reproductive Health: New Perspectives on Men's Participation (vol. 26, no. 2, October 1998), series J, no. 46.

Ending Violence against Women (vol. 27, no. 4, December 1999), series L, no. 11.

Meeting the Needs of Young Adults (vol. 23, no. 3, October 1995).

Controlling Sexually Transmitted Diseases (vol. 21, no. 1, June 1993).

Tel.: 410-659-6300; Fax: 410-659-6266; E-mail: *Poprepts@jhuccp.org; www.jhuccp.org*

—

The Clearinghouse on Infant Feeding and Maternal Nutrition produces a regular free newsletter of abstracts on infant feeding relevant to developing countries. For more information contact: American Public Health Association Clearinghouse, 1015 15th Street N.W., Washington, DC 20005, USA. Tel.: 202-777-2463; Fax: 202-777-2534; E-mail: *apha@permanet.org; aphach@igc.apc.org.*

WEBSITES

ACT UP (*www.actup.org*) ACT UP is a diverse, nonpartisan group of individuals united in anger and committed to direct action to end the AIDS crisis.

AIDS Education Global Information System (AEGIS): *www.aegis.com*

The Body website: *www.thebody.com.* This page is written for people who have just found out that they are HIV-positive and provides much information that is both useful and comforting. The Body is a U.S. website, so much of the practical information on where to find help is aimed at North Americans. The site also has Spanish information.

Centers for Disease Control and Prevention: Division of HIV/AIDS Prevention (DHAP). *www.cdc.gov.* The CDC's HIV mission is to prevent HIV infection and reduce the incidence of HIV-related illness and death, in collaboration with community, state, national, and international partners.

Drum Beat (*www.comminit.com*) This is an e-mail and web network from THE COMMUNICATION INITIATIVE partnership with The Rockefeller Foundation, UNICEF, USAID, WHO, BBC World Service, CIDA, Johns Hopkins Center for Communication Programs, Soul City, The Panos Institute, and UNFPA. It offers information, ideas, and dialogue on communication, development, and change, including sexual health and HIV/AIDS issues.

ELDIS (*www.ids.ac.uk*) ELDIS, a Gateway to Information Sources on Development and the Environment, offers an easy route to the latest information on development and environmental issues as both a directory and an entry point to electronic information resources. It is available free via the Internet. Recent new entries related to HIV/AIDS include materials on World Bank Health Sector Reforms and on gender and health.

The Global Network of people living with HIV/AIDS (GNP+) (*www.hivnet.ch*) is a global network for and by people with HIV/AIDS. The central secretariat of the network is based in Amsterdam, Netherlands, and has a board of twelve members.

The International AIDS Vaccine Initiative's (IAVI) mission is to ensure the development of safe, effective, accessible, preventive HIV vaccines for use throughout the world. IAVI's website provides information about IAVI's activities and background information and news about AIDS vaccine development.

Inventory of Applied Health Research in Emergency Settings. International Health Unit, Macfarlane Burnet Institute for Medical Research and Public Health. Melbourne: MBC/WHO/EHA, 2000 (*community@ burnet.edu.au*).

The ProCAARE e-mail discussion forum on all aspects of HIV/AIDS, established as a partnership between SatelLife and the Harvard AIDS Institute/Harvard School of Public Health (HAI), has been operating since 1996. To participate in discussions on ProCAARE, send a message to *procaare@usa .healthnet.org*. You must always give your full name, affiliation, and physical address when you submit a message. ProCAARE discussions are archived and the archives can be searched at *www.healthnet.org*.

Sexually Transmitted Infections (*www.who.int.*) This WHO Communicable Disease Surveillance and Response site includes information on HIV/AIDS and sexually transmitted infections as well as links to many other AIDS-related sites.

Straight Talk Foundation (useful for IEC materials), PO Box 22366, Kampala, Uganda. *Strtalk@swiftuganda .com*.

Strategies for Hope Series *www.stratshope.org*. — Strategies for Hope is a series of books and videos which focus mainly on sub-Saharan Africa, and also includes the training package "Stepping Stones." Issues covered include counseling, home-based care, workplace-based prevention, orphans, young people, and gender issues.

UNAIDS: *www.unaids.org*.

REFERENCE ADDRESSES

Centers for Disease Control and Prevention
International Emergency and Refugee Health Branch,
Mailstop F-48, 4770 Buford Highway
Atlanta, GA 30341 USA
Fax: 770-488-7829
Website: *www.cdc.gov*

Healthlink Worldwide
Cityside, 40 Adler Street, London E1 1EE, UK
Fax 44-20-7539-1580; *Publications@healthlink.org.uk*
www.healthink.org.uk

International Federation of the Red Cross and Red Crescent Societies
17, Chemin des Crets, Case postale 372
1211 Geneva, Switzerland
Fax: 41-22-730-0395; Website: *www.ifrc.org*

International Rescue Committee
Health Unit, 122 East 42nd Street, New York, NY 10168
Tel.: 212-551-3000; Fax: 212-551-3185
Website: *www.theirc.org*.

International Planned Parenthood Federation
Regent's College Inner Circle, London NW1 4NS UK
Fax: 44-20-7847-7950; Website: *www.ippf.org*

Médecins Sans Frontières International
39, rue de la Tourelle, B-1040 Brussels, Belgium
Fax: 32-2-474-7575; Website: *www.msf.org*

Population Information Program
Johns Hopkins School of Public Health
111 Market Street, Suite 310, Baltimore, MD 21202 USA
Fax: 410-659-6266;
E-mail: *poprepts@welchlink.welch.jhu.edu*

Reproductive Health for Refugees Consortium (RHR Consortium)
Contact: The Women's Commission for Refugee Women and Children, 122 East 42nd Street, 12th Floor, New York, NY 10168 USA
Fax: 212-551-3186; Website: *www.rhrc.org*
E-mail: *wcrwc@intrescom.org*

Save the Children Fund UK
17 Grove Lane, London SE5 8RD UK
Fax: 44-20-7703-2275

TALC (Teaching Aids at Low Cost)
PO Box 49, St Albans, Herts AL1 5TX UK
Fax: 44-1727-846-852; *talcuk@btinternet.com*
www.talcuk.org

UNAIDS, Information Centre
1211 Geneva 27, Switzerland
Fax: 41-22-791-4187; E-mail: *unaids@unaids.org*
www.unaids.org

UNFPA
Contact local country offices or
220 East 42nd Street, New York, NY 10017 USA
Fax: 212-297-4915

UNFPA Emergency Relief Office
9 Chemin des Anemones, 1219 Geneva, Switzerland
Fax: 41-22-979-9049; E-mail: *unfpaero@undp.org*
Website: *www.unfpa.org*

UNHCR — Centre for Documentation for Refugees
Case postale 2500, 1211 Geneva 2 Switzerland
Fax: 41-22-739-8111; E-mail: *cdr@unhcr.ch*
Website: *www.unhcr.org*

UNICEF
Three United Nations Plaza, New York, NY 10017 USA
Fax: 212-824-6464; Website: *www.unicef.org*

World Health Organization
Distribution and Sales
1211 Geneva 27 Switzerland
E-mail: *publications@who.ch*

World Health Organization
Department of Reproductive Health and Research
1211 Geneva 27 Switzerland
Fax: 41-22-791-4189;
E-mail: *reproductivehealth@who.int*
Website: *www.who.org*

World Bank
1818 H Street N.W., Washington, DC 20433 USA
Fax: 202-477-6391; Website: *www.worldbank.org*

REGIONAL NETWORKS
OF PEOPLE LIVING WITH HIV/AIDS

Asia Pacific Network of People Living with HIV and AIDS
84 Woo Mon Chew Road, Singapore 455160
Tel.: 65-6448-5958; Fax: 65-6446-2916
E-mail: *apn@pacific.net.sg*

Caribbean Regional Network of People Living with HIV/AIDS
P.O. Bag 133, St. James, Port of Spain, Trinidad, W.I.
Voice mail: 868-622-8045; Tel./Fax: 868-622-0176
E-mail: *crn@carib-link.net*

European Network of Positive People
250 Kennington Lane, London SE11 5RD, England
Tel.: 44-20-7564-2180; Fax: 44-20-7564-2140
E-mail: *ikramer@ukcoalition.demon.co.uk*

GNP+ North America
2-12 Seaman Ave, 3H, New York, NY 10034, USA
Tel.: 212-569-6023; Fax: 212-942-8530
E-mail: *babaluaye@aol.com*

Latin American Network of People Living with HIV/AIDS
CC 117 Suc. 2 "B" (1402), Buenos Aires, Argentina
Tel./Fax: 5411-4807-2772 E-mail: *jihb@pinos.com*

Network of African People Living with HIV and AIDS
P.O. Box 32717, Lusaka, Zambia
Tel.: 260-1-223-191/151; Fax: 260-1-223-209
E-mail: *napnzp@zamnet.zm*

UNAIDS: focal person for the greater involvement of people living with HIV/AIDS (GIPA): Salvator Niyonzima, Department of Policy, Strategy and Research,
20, Avenue Appia, CH-1211 Geneva 27, Switzerland
Tel.: 41-22-791-4448; Fax: 41-22-791-4741
E-mail: *niyonzimas@unaids.org*

Index

Underlined page references indicate figures.

Acquired Immune Deficiency Syndrome. *See* AIDS *and AIDS-related listings.*
action, as stage of change, 86
ActionAid, 115
Aga Khan Health Network, 43
AIDS, 19
  acceptance of diagnosis, 75
  case definition, 21
  cause of, 21
  difficulty in understanding, 72
  infections and cancers accompanying, 20
  information materials, 100–101
  low priority for displaced and conflict-affected populations, 74
  prognosis, 21
  symptoms in final stages, 21, 178
AIDS Action newsletter, 33
AIDS cases, notification of, 42–43
AIDS counseling awareness workshop, 70
AIDS education, 109
AIDSline database, 39
The AIDS Support Organization. *See* TASO
alcohol, role in spread of HIV, 10
amniocentesis, increased HIV risk from, 24
anal sex, method of HIV transmission, 22
animal milk, 145
anonymous testing, voluntary, 42
antibody tests, 90
antiretroviral drugs, 25, 146, 182–83, 184
antiretroviral prophylaxis (ARVP), 141, 150, 173
APN+ (Asia Pacific Network of People Living with HIV/AIDS), 133
appeal, in communication campaign, 104–6
attitude change, through community communication activities, 115–17
attributable risk, 10
autologous blood transfusion, 163–64
awareness-raising days, 104
AZT, 141

babies
  feeding, 142. *See also* breast-feeding *and breast-feeding related entries*
  HIV infection in, 155
baby-friendly hospitals, 144, 187

bacterial vaginosis, 23, 96
barrier nursing, 167
barriers wall, 204, <u>205</u>
behavior change, 85–86
  communication materials for, 100–107
  counseling, 67
  enabling environment for, 86–87
  legal framework, 86
  religious factors, 86
  social factors, 86
bereavement counseling scenarios, 77
bias, in quantitative surveys, 44
blood, bacterial infection of, 182
blood banks, 159
blood screening
  linked vs. unlinked, 162, 163
  reducing costs of, 162–63
blood splashes, 23, 167–68
blood testing, 159
blood transfusion
  donor selection guidelines, 160–62
  encouraging use of autologous transfusion, 162–64
  establishing routine blood screening, 162–63
  indicators and methods of measurement, <u>165</u>
  method of contracting HIV, 23
  micro transfusions, 160
  preventing transmission through, 159
  reducing, 160
  risk of HIV with, 10
  strict criteria for, 159–60, <u>161</u>
body mapping, 47
Botswana, 92
breast-feeding
  avoiding, 141
  balancing the risks, 143
  benefits, 142
  in counseling on HIV and infant feeding, 152–54
  exclusive, 3, 24, 142, 143, 153
  modifying, 142–43
  replacement options, 143–45
  risk of HIV transmission with, 23, 24, 153–54
  steps for success, 144
  supporting mothers, 145
brochures, 102
buprenorphine, 128

caesarean section
  effect on HIV risk, 24
  elective, 141–42
candida albicans, syndromic management, <u>211</u>
candidiasis, 23
caregivers, care and support for
  arranging, 188
  indicators and methods of measurement, <u>191</u>
causal diagram, 204
causal pathway for planning, 58, <u>59</u>, <u>60</u>
CD4 count, 182
Center for Disease Control and Prevention, 21
chancroid, syndromic management, 208, <u>213</u>, <u>214</u>
checklists, counseling, 77, 79–81, 152–54
childbirth, questions for situation analysis regarding
    knowledge, beliefs, and practice, 196
children
  counseling for, 75–76
  HIV infection symptoms in, 139
chlamydia, 96, 207, <u>208</u>, <u>209</u>, <u>212</u>
church groups, 105
circumcision, lack of, risk of HIV, 23
clinic care, indicators and methods of measurement,
    <u>190</u>
communication, 100, 101
communication campaigns
  appeal, 104–6
  channels for, 102–4
  choosing terminology carefully, 106
  community activities, 115–17
  evaluating response to, 106
  message content, 101–2
  pre-testing materials and ideas, 106
  production and distribution, 106
communication opportunities, questions for situation
    analysis, 194
"community," defining for refugee/IDP population, 55
community counseling, 104
community development initiatives, 110
community education, blood donation, 160
community health status, questions for situation
    analysis, 194
condoms
  accepting use of, 86
  attitude towards, 91–92, 93
  Catholics reluctant to promote use of, 95
  female, 23, 92–93
  formula for calculating requirements, 95
  increasing accessibility, 94
  instructing on use of, 95, 96, <u>97</u>
  male, 23, 92
  prevention against HIV infection, 14
  promotion and distribution, 84, 93–95, 101, <u>119</u>
  question guide (theme list) for use of, <u>49</u>

confidentiality
  difficulty in pregnancy or post-partum period, 147
  importance of, 50, 51, 70, 71
  shared, 67
  training on importance of, 70
confirmatory tests, 90–91
conflict-affected populations, loss of sense of control,
    85
consultation, 51
contact tracing, 99–100
contaminated waste, 171
contemplation, as stage of change, 85–86
continuum of care, 175–76
controversial issues, addressing, 3
Convention Relating to the Status of Refugees, 57
counseling
  checklists for, 77, 152–54
  for children, 75–76
  community, 104
  crisis, 75, 77
  defined, 67
  group, 146
  indicators for, <u>82</u>
  infant feeding and HIV, 143–46, 152–54
  during information-gathering process, 51
  measuring effects of, 69
  post-test, 72–73, 76–77, <u>80–81</u>
  pre-test, 70–72, 76, <u>79</u>, 147
  prevention, 69, 75
  problem-solving, 73–75
  rape victims and HIV, 114
  rationale for, 68–69
  role-plays, 76, 92
  scenarios, 76–77
  selecting trainees for, 69–70
  services, voluntary, 43
  skills needed, 68, 69
  strategies for, 69–77
  suitable venues, 68
  support for counselors, 77–78
  supportive, 73–75, 181
  training counselors, 69–70
  training exercise, 76
  types of, 67
  useful situations for, 67
  voluntary, 69
counselors
  qualities for, 68
  selecting trainees for, 69–70
  support for, 77–78
  training, 69–70, 134
couple visit, with HIV-positive pregnant spouse, 147
cow's milk formula, 145

crisis counseling, 67, 75
  during post-test counseling, 73
  scenarios, 77
cross-sectional surveys, 42

data collection
  quantitative methods, 42–44
  tools, 44–47
dead body, contamination from, 169
decision-making counseling, 67
decision-making structures, questions for situation
  analysis, 193
decontamination methods, <u>169</u>
Democratic Republic of the Congo, 149
De Montfort incinerator, 171
demographic data, questions for situation analysis, 193
denial, 70, 74
dependents, coordinating care and support for, 188–89
depressants, 124
diagnosis, acceptance of, 75
discharge policy, 183
discussion sessions, 9
displaced populations
  loss of sense of control, 85
  vulnerable to rapid spread of infections, 1
displacement
  consequences of, 29–31
  effect on attitudes toward pregnancy, 83
  facilitating spread of HIV and STIs, 29, 31
  impact on sexual practices and attitudes, 83–84
domestic violence, 111
DOTS (Directly Observed Therapy Short course), 107,
  181
drugs, injecting, 123, 169
  advocacy and stigma reduction, 126–27
  drugs commonly used, 123–24
  drug treatment programs, 127–28
  education and communication, 125–26
  harm prevention, 124
  harm reduction, 129
  questions for situation analysis, 196
  reasons for, 126
  transmission prevention rationale, 124
  transmission prevention strategies, 124–28
drugs, for PLWH/A care, 183
drug substitution, 128
drug treatment, for PLWH/A, 184
drug use, indicators and measurement methods, <u>130</u>
drug users, selling blood, 160
dry sex, 23, 109

Eastern Europe, increasing HIV epidemic, 24
Eastern Zaire, 93

education, 100, 101
effect indicators, 60
ELISA (Enzyme Linked Immuno-Sorbent Assay), 27,
  90, 162, 163
elites, questions for situation analysis, 193
Epi-info, 44
episiotomy, effect on HIV risk, 24
ethical framework, developing, 3–4
evaluation, 58–60
  making fun and interesting, 62
  timing of, 59–60
exercise, 177
exercises
  gathering sensitive information, 201–5
  gender expectations, group discussion, 15
  HIV epidemic, 13–14
  role-play training, 76
  sexuality and sexual health group discussion,
    15–16
  Stepping Stones, 115–17
  transmission picture card game, 10–12
exposure, accidental, 171, 173

faith-based networks, 86
false negatives, 91
false positives, 27, 89–90, 91
fathers, postnatal counseling, 149
female condom, 92–93
fermentation, 177
flip charts, 102
florid pulmonary tuberculosis, 182
flow diagrams, 47
focus group discussions, 41, 44–45
  filming, 62–63
  third-person approach, 49
folk media, 103–4
former Soviet Union, increasing HIV epidemic, 24

gender analysis, 4
gender expectations, group discussion exercise, 15
gender relations, 112, 193
gender roles, displacement's effect on, 29
gender violence
  Burundian refugees in Tanzania, 40
  new emphasis on, 2
  preventing and managing consequences of, 110–12
genital herpes, 208–9
gonorrhea, 96, 98, 207, <u>208</u>, <u>209</u>, <u>212</u>
grief counseling, 67
group counseling, 146
Guidelines for HIV Interventions in Emergency Settings
  (UNAIDS), 2

harm reduction strategies, drug injecting, 124, <u>125,</u> 126, 129

health care, access to and use of, questions for situation analysis, 194

health care service activities

developing policies and protocols, 186

establishing home-based care system, 187

prioritizing care and support, 186

training health care staff, 187

health care settings

indicators and methods of measurement, <u>174</u>

preventing transmission in, 167, 172

health care workers

HIV-infected, 171–72

lack of HIV information among, 133, 168

hepatitis B, 21, 23, 124, 168

hepatitis C, 23, 124, 168

heterosexual sex, risk of HIV with, 10

high prevalence population, 90

high-risk behavior groups

difficulty in reaching, 39

targeting interventions at, 84

HIV

addressing in different contexts, 2

AIDS as final stage of infection, 20

antibody testing, purposes of, 22

antibody testing, reliability of, 27

babies born to infected mothers, 26

blood level high immediately after infection, 23

challenges to prevention, care, and support in displacement and conflict settings, 2–4

checking knowledge of, 17

commonly asked questions, 25–27

counseling checklist for infant feeding, 152–54

defined, 19

diagnosis and staging, 181–82

difficulty diagnosing in infants, 139

discussing possibility of with a partner, 71

easier transmission in presence of other STIs, 96

epidemiology and surveillance, 24

exercise demonstrating rapid spread of, 13–14

existing activities to prevent spread of, 3

fluids virus is present in, 167

growing awareness of, 2

human rights framework for addressing spread and impact of, 57

impact of epidemic on refugee/IDP population, 31

infection of babies, 155

infection during pregnancy or post-partum period, 146

infection in partners, 26

interventions in health care settings, 172

isolation of people infected with, 25

killed by heat, 19, 145, 169

lack of knowledge about one's own status, 14

latency, 19–20

limited information among health professionals, 133, 168

MISP activities to reduce transmission, 35

mother-child transmission increased in presence of STI, 100

myths about, 21

neurological and psychiatric complications affecting behavior, 74

NGOs' role in response to, 33–34

pattern of transmission in populations forced to migrate, 24

primary prevention, 140

prophylactic medicines for, 25

public disclosure of positive status, 39

rapid course of disease in infants, 139

reducing risk of infection through transfusion, 159

reducing vulnerability to, 33

review of existing data, 39–40

risk of occupational transmission, 167–68

risk of transmission with breast-feeding, 153–54

secondary prevention, 141

source of, 25

stages of infection, 19–20

STIs increasing risk of contracting and transmitting, 22–23

strategic planning for prevention and care, 35–36

studies of prevalence, 42–43

symptoms, 19–20, 139

test-dependent interventions for MTCT, 141–43

test results for, 27

therapies and treatment, 20

threat of a low priority for refugees and IDPs, 2–3

time to AIDS infection, 20

transmission methods, 22–24

treatment for, 25

understanding vulnerability to, 29, <u>30</u>

vaccine for, 26

vulnerability to and choice of interventions, 56–58

waiting for test result, 14

HIV-1, 19, 162

HIV-2, 19, 162

HIV/AIDS, estimated population living with, <u>20</u>

HIV antibody tests, interpreting results, 89–90

HIV education, constraints and frustrations, 4

HIV epidemic

exercise, 13–14

measures taken in acute emergency phase and afterward, 1

HIV infection

frequency and distribution, questions for situation analysis, 194

tests for, 21

HIV intervention
    importance of consultation in refugee/IDP communities, 34
    men not engaged in, 4
    situation analysis, 34
HIV prevention and care
    coordination with other sectors, 3
    counseling for, 67
    first steps in, 7
    incorporating into existing programs, 33
    integrating with existing activities, 2
    strategic planning process for, 55–63
HIV prevention, key features contributing to, 84
HIV response review, 35–36, 38
HIV situation analysis, 35–36
    information-gathering methods, 38
    outsiders' role in, 39
    topics of interest, 37–38
HIV strategies
    planning, 37–38
    selection and prioritizing factors, 37
    testing, 199–200
HIV tests
    advantages and disadvantages, 71–72, 89
    choosing, 91
    types of, 90–91
    virus tests, 91
HIV training, transmission picture card game, 10–12
home-based care, 176–79
    establishing, 187–88
    indicators and methods of measurement, 190
    kits, 188
home-based carers, infection control training, home nursing care, 177–78
home visits, for HIV education, STI treatment, and condom distribution, 3
Hong Kong, 129
hospital care
    indicators and methods of measurement, 190
    for PLWH/A, 181–83
hospitals, PLWH friendly, 187
Human Immunodeficiency Virus. *See* HIV *and HIV-related listings*
humanitarian agencies
    development activities after crisis period, 2
    role in addressing HIV epidemic, 1–2
human rights framework, 3–4, 57
hygiene behavior, 105

IDP (internally displaced persons), new emphasis on reproductive health needs, 2
IDP community
    characteristics of, 29
    potential harm from information-gathering, 50–51

IEC (Information, Education, and Communication), 100
    campaign, for PTCT, 151
    materials, indicators and methods of measurement, 120
illustrations, 103
impact indicators, 60–61
income-generating activities, 117
in-depth interviews, 45–46
India, 24, 139
indicators, 60–62
    blood transfusions, 165
    caregiver care, 191
    choosing, 61–62
    clinic care, 190
    drug use, 130
    health care settings, 174
    home-based care, 190
    hospital care, 190
    orphan support, 191
    PLWH/A, 135
    PTCT issues, 156
    sexual violence, 117–18
    SMART, 62
    STIs, 117–18
infant feeding, questions for situation analysis regarding knowledge, beliefs, and practice, 196–97
Infant Feeding in Emergencies, 143
infection control practices, 170
infertility, concern for refugees and IDPs, 3
information, 100, 101
information-gathering
    ethical considerations, 50–52
    participatory approach to, 38–39
    presenting findings, 52
    process, 38–39
    qualitative methods, 38, 44–50
    quantitative methods, 38, 42–44
information sessions, 9
informed consent, 51, 70, 71, 88, 146–47, 181
injecting drug use, 23, 123. *See also* drugs
integrating programs for various concerns, 3
Inter-Agency Manual of Reproductive Health in Refugee Settings, 112
Inter-Agency Task Force, 151
interest groups, questions for situation analysis, 193
internally displaced persons. *See* IDP *and related IDP listings*
International AIDS vaccine initiative, 26
International Narcotics Control Board, 178
interventions, 58
    changing individual behaviors, 87, 100–110
    choosing indicators for, 61–62
    framework for planning, 87

interventions (continued)
  provision of services, 87–100
  sexual violence prevention, 113
  sexual violence response, 113
  societal context, 87, 110–17
  test-dependent for PTCT, 150
interviews
  distinguishing between counseling session and
    research interview, 51
  tips, 45–46
intraoperative blood salvage, 164
IRC (International Rescue Committee), 39, 40, 58, 116,
  149
*IRC Guide to Program Planning and Proposal Development: Effective Design, Monitoring, and Evaluation
  of IRC Projects in the Field Operations Manual,*
  59
isolation practices, 167

Kaleeba, Noerine, 147
Kenya, 111

lactation
  HIV contracted during, 24
  preventing new infections during, 148
leaflets, 102
legal issues, questions for situation analysis, 197
literacy programs, 3, 33
literate clients, providing printed information to, 73
low prevalence population, 90

magazines, 102
maintenance, as stage of change, 86
male condom, 92. *See also* condoms
mandatory testing, 88
man's right to information, with pregnant, HIV-positive
  spouse, 147
mapping, 47
mass media, 102
matrix ranking, 48
measurement, methods for
  blood transfusions, <u>165</u>
  caregiver care, <u>191</u>
  clinic care, <u>190</u>
  drug use, <u>130</u>
  health care settings, 174
  home-based care, <u>190</u>
  hospital care, <u>190</u>
  orphan support, <u>191</u>
  PLWH/A, <u>135</u>
  PTCT issues, <u>156</u>
Médecins Sans Frontières, 129
medicines, for symptom management, 177

Medline database, 39
Memory Books Programme, 183–85
men
  involving in reproductive health programs, 4
  reaching with sexual behavior change programs, 84
  unengaged in HIV interventions, 4
methadone maintenance, 128
microbicide, 93
microfinance programs, 117
midwives
  practices, effect on HIV risk, 24
  risk to, 168
miliary tuberculosis, 182
MISP (Minimum Initial Service Package), 34, 35, 93,
  111
monitoring and evaluation, defined, 58
moral messages, mixing with health messages, 105
morphine, 179
Mosedame, Billy, 175
mosquitos, 26
mouth-to-mouth resuscitation, 169
Mozambique, 96
MTCT (mother-to-child transmission), 23–24, 139
  care for the mother, 147–48

*National AIDS Programmes: A Guide to Monitoring
  and Evaluation,* 59
National Blood Transfusion Service, 159
needle-stick injuries, 23, 167–68, 173
needle-syringe programs. *See* NSPs
negative test result
  post-test counseling, 73, <u>81</u>, 88
  strategies for, 199–200
networks, questions for situation analysis, 193
neurological disease, 182
nevirapine, 141, 146
New Emergency Health Kit, 178, 179
newsletters, 102
newspapers, 102
NGOs
  role in response to HIV, 33–34
  staff, characteristics of, 9
  variety of venues operating in, 2
non-governmental organizations. *See* NGOs
NSPs, 124, 127
nutritional support, 177
Nutrition for Developing Countries, 143

observation, as qualitative information-gathering
  method, 47
occupational exposures, reporting and managing, 172
occupational transmission, 167–68
100 Percent Condom Program, 84

Opening Up the HIV Epidemic: Guidance on Encouraging Beneficial Disclosure, Ethical Partner Counseling, and Appropriate Use of HIV Case Reporting, 71
opiates, 123
opportunistic infections, 181, 182
    managing, 179
    treatment for, 25
organ transplant, method of contracting HIV, 23
orphaned children, 140
    care and support for, 183–86
    coordinating care and support for, 188–89
    indicators and methods of measuring support, 191
outpatient cards, 185
output indicators, 60
outreach, 84
Oxfam, 41

pain management, 178–79
palliative care, 178
parent-to-child transmission. *See* PTCT
Paris AIDS Summit Declaration, 132
participatory action research, 46
participatory appraisal exercises, 46–47, 48
participatory learning and action (PLA), 115
    exercises, 41, 45, 46–47, 201–5
participatory rural appraisal, 46
partner notification, 99–100
peer education, 86, 106–7
    among drug injectors, 125
    IEC materials helpful in, 101
    stigmatization of, 107–8
peer strategies, 84
peer support, for PLWH/A, 133
picture code, 103
PLWH/A (people living with HIV/AIDS), 175
    acceptance of, 69
    building capacity and enhancing skills of, 133–34
    care and support for, questions for situation analysis, 195
    drugs for, 25
    home-based care for, 176–79
    increased support for, 86
    indicators and methods of measurement, 135
    peer support groups, 133
    perception of, 131
    personalizing risk of disease, 109
    possible contributions of, 131–32
    primary health care for, 179–81
    protecting human rights of, 133
    regional networks, 218
    resentment of term, 131 n.1
    respecting rights of, 131
    role in prevention activities, 110
    self-care, 176
    stigma associated with, 132–33
    training counselors for, 134
    as volunteer carers, 188
PLWH-friendly hospitals, 187
political conflicts, long-lasting nature of, 2
Population Services International, 94
positive test results, 70
    post-test counseling, 81, 88
    reactions to, 73
    strategies for, 199–200
    telling partner about, 73
post-emergency phase, care and support activities, 186
posters, 3, 33, 102–3
post-partum period
    increased risk of transmission during, 140
    infection during, 146
    preventing new infections during, 148
post-test counseling, 67, 72–73, 76–77, 80–81, 88
    including information on PLWH/A peer support, 133
    related to screening blood for transfusion, 162, 163
    scenarios, 76–77
poverty, major reason for HIV vulnerability, 21, 117
precontemplation, as stage of change, 85–86
pregnancy
    attitudes toward affected by displacement, 83
    increased risk of transmission during, 140
    infection during, 146
    knowledge, beliefs, and practice, questions for situation analysis, 196
    method of passing along HIV, 23–24
    preventing new infections during, 148
    testing and screening during, 146
pregnant women, concerns of regarding HIV, 139–40
prenatal testing, informed consent, 146
preparation, as stage of change, 86
pre-test counseling, 67, 70–72, 76, 79, 88, 147
    scenarios, 76
    related to screening blood for transfusion, 162
prevention
    primary, 98, 140, 157
    secondary, 98, 141, 148–50, 157
prevention counseling, 67, 75, 69, 99, 110
    scenarios, 77
primary health care, 179–81
Primary Health Care Management Advancement Programme (PHCMAP), 43
primary prevention, PTCT, 157
print media, 102–3
prioritizing care and support activities, 186
problem aunties, 109–10
problem-solving counseling, 73–75
prophylactic medicines, 25
prophylaxis, 180

protective equipment, for health care workers, 172

provision of services, indicators and methods of measurement, 119

PTCT (parent-to-child transmission), 139

  conceptualizing prevention of HIV transmission, 157

  counselor training, 150

  IEC community campaign, 151

  impacts of, 139–40

  integrating strategies with maternal and reproductive health work, 149

  issues regarding, indicators and methods of measurement, 156

  prevention, primary, 140, 157

  prevention, secondary, 141, 157

  prevention and care strategies, 148

  test-dependent interventions, 150

puppet shows, 103

qualitative methods, 38, 44–50

  data analysis, 48–50

  planning for, 47–48

quantitative methods, 38, 42–44

question guides, preparing, 48

questionnaire surveys, 43–44

radio, 102

ranking, 47, 48

rape

  economics and, 112

  increased likelihood of, 111

  men affected by, 29, 111

  protection from, 1, 33

  support for victims of, 50, 70, 83

  worries about HIV after, 174

rapid appraisal methods, reproductive health issues, 41

rapid testing, 42, 146–47

referral systems, 181

refugees, new emphasis on reproductive health needs, 2

religious messages, 104, 105

religious organizations, 105

Reproductive Health in Refugee Situations Field Manual, 4

reproductive health services, 148–50

  involving men in, 4

resources

  behavior change, 121

  blood transfusions, 164

  care-giving, 192

  communication, 121

  condoms, 121

  counseling, 78

  drug use, 128

  education for health care workers, 172

  HIV basic facts, 27

  how-to guides for reproductive health in refugee situations, 63

  Lessons Learned series, 63–64

  manuals and guidelines, 215–16

  newsletters, 216

  PLWH/A, 134

  PTCT issues, 158

  sexual violence and coerced sex, 122

  STI management and control, 121

  strategic planning process, 63

  voluntary counseling and testing, 121

  websites, 216–17

  youth, 121–22

respite care, 179

response review, planning guide, 52–53

risk matrix, 58

role-plays, 47, 76

Rwanda, 116

safer sexual practices, 9, 83

sampling, for rapid community surveys, 43–44

seasonal calendar, 47

secondary prevention

  interventions, 148–50

  PTCT, 157

Senegal, 84, 86

sentinel surveillance, 24, 42

seroconversion, 19, 79

sex

  importance of dialoguing about, 9

  most common route of HIV transmission, 83

sex education, for young people, 108–10

sex toys, 23

sexual abuse, 111

sexual activity, roughness and frequency increasing likelihood of spreading HIV, 23

sexual behavior patterns, questions for situation analysis, 195–96

sexual health, 108–9

  group discussion exercise, 15–16

  WHO definition of, 16, 108

sexual partner, exclusive, 14

sexual practices and attitude, impact of displacement on, 83

sexual violence

  Burundian refugees in Tanzania, 40

  indicators, 117–18

  interventions for prevention and response, 113

  new emphasis on, 2

  prevention and care provision for survivors, indicators and methods of measurement, 120

  preventing and managing consequences of, 110–12

  protecting women from, 3

sexuality, group discussion exercise, 15–16

sexually transmitted infections. *See STI listings*

sex work, helping women avoid, 3

sex workers

　involving in research, 39

　as peer educators, 63

simple/rapid assay, 163

situation analysis

　planning guide, 52–53

　providing baseline information, 62

　questions to assist in planning for, 193–97

social activities, 112–15

social events, 104

social marketing, 94, 99

societal context, interventions related to, 110–17

socioeconomic data, questions for situation analysis, 193

Southeast Asia, 24, 139

Stages of Change Model, 85–86

standard precautions. *See* universal precautions

Stepping Stones, 115–17

sterilization, 169–71

stigmatization

　associated with HIV infection, 33, 103, 105

　of behaviors and practices, 3, 34

　against caregivers, 188

　with counseling, 68, 71

　drug use, 126–27

　of high-risk groups, 84, 101

　of peer educators, 108

　of PLWH/A, 37, 56, 71, 106, 131–33

　of people with STIs, 98

stimulants, 123

STIs (sexually transmitted infections)

　causes of rapid spread, 1

　common, 96

　concern for refugees and IDPs, 3

　correct diagnosis, 98–99

　early detection, 100

　effects of, 96

　encouraging care-seeking behavior, 100

　frequency and distribution, questions for situation analysis, 194

　improving access to treatment, 98

　incidence of, 96

　increasing risk of contracting and transmitting HIV, 22–23

　indicators, 117–18

　prevention counseling, 99

　prevention and management, indicators and methods of measuring, <u>119</u>

　primary prevention, 98

　rapid spread among displaced populations, 1

　secondary prevention, 98

　strategic planning for prevention and care, 35–36

　strengthening management and control of, 96–100

　surveillance, 100

　syndromic management, 99, <u>207</u>, 207–14

　treatment, 99

　ulcerative, 22

strategic planning, for monitoring and evaluation

　causal pathway for, 58

　choosing interventions, 56–58

　detailed planning, 58

　guiding principles, 55–56

　identifying gaps in response to problems, 56

　including different perspectives, 62

　indicators, 60–62

　participation in, 62–63

　problem definition, 56

Suaudeau, Jacques, 95

sub-Saharan Africa, 24, 96, 139, 160

Sudan, appraising reproductive health needs in, 41

supplies, needed in hospital setting for PLWH/A care, 183

supportive counseling, 67, 73–75, 181

surgeons, risk to, 168

surveillance, 24, 100

survey participants, potential harm to, 50

survey planning, 43

syphilis, 96, 98, 100, 207, <u>213</u>, <u>214</u>

Tanzania, 40, 85, 96

target groups, for communication campaigns, 101

TASO (The AIDS Support Organization), 69, 70

ten seed technique, 48, 204

test-dependent interventions, limitations of, 146

testing

　anonymous, 42

　antibody, 22

　during pregnancy, 146

　HIV strategies, 199

　mandatory, 43, 88

　prenatal, 146

　rapid, 42, 146–47

　voluntary services, 43

Thailand, 84, 141

thrush, 23

time-lines, 47

tissue transplant, method of contracting HIV, 23

traditional healers, 181

The Training Guide to IRC's Program Design, Monitoring, and Evaluation Framework, 59

transactional sex, 16, 195

transfusions, complete, 27

transmission picture card game, 10–12

trichomonas, 98, <u>211</u>

tuberculosis, 180–81

Uganda, 84, 99, 141, 183
UNAIDS, 71, 94
    assistance with blood screening, 163
    counseling defined, 67
    existing data on HIV prevalence, 39
    guidelines on infant feeding and HIV, 143, 144
    HIV epidemic classifications, 24
    HIV testing strategies, 199
    strategic planning guide, 35
UNAIDS Policy on HIV Testing and Counseling, 88
UN Commission on Human Rights, 111
UNDP
    linking NGOs with microfinance institutions, 117
    Human Development Report, 39
UNFPA, 94
UNHCR, 94, 111
    Guidelines for Prevention and Response to Sexual
        Violence against Refugees, 111
    Protection Guidelines, 113
UNICEF, 39
    Baby-Friendly Hospital initiative, 144
    guidelines on infant feeding and HIV, 143, 144
Universal Declaration of Human Rights, 57
universal infection control precautions, 23, 170, 133,
        168, 169, 170, 172
unmarried staff, presumption of no sexual experience, 9
unsafe sex, protection from, 3
UN Security Guidelines for Women, 113
unwanted pregnancy, concern for refugees and IDPs, 3

vaccine, 26
vaginal discharge with speculum, syndromic
        management, 210
vaginal sexual intercourse
    method of HIV transmission, 22, 23
    risk of HIV with, 10
VCT (voluntary counseling and testing), 69, 87–91, 92,
        175
    prenatal, 141
    services, indicators and methods of measurement,
        119
visual electric media, 104

voluntary counseling and testing. *See* VCT
volunteer care, 177

welfare services, questions for situation analysis,
        194
Western Blot confirmatory test, 90, 163, 199
wet-nurses, 145
WHO, 39, 71, 94
    addressing narcotics availability, 178, 179
    assistance with blood screening, 163
    Baby-Friendly Hospital initiative, 144
    categories of HIV clinical status, 182
    Clinical Management of Survivors of Rape, 114
    definition of sexual health, 16, 108
    field manual on tuberculosis control in refugee/IDP
        settings, 180
    guidelines for clinical diagnosis of AIDS in adults, 21,
        22
    guidelines on infant feeding and HIV-infected
        mothers, 143, 144
    HIV testing strategies, 199
    nevirapine approved, 141
    "Operational Characteristics of Commercially
        Available Assays to Determine Antibodies to HIV-1
        and/or HIV-2 in Human Sera," 91
    protocols for survivors of sexual violence, 113
    strategies for confirming positive HIV antibody test,
        90
widow cleansing, 117
window period, 21, 23, 79, 88
World Bank, 39
World Health Assembly, 178
World Health Organization. *See* WHO

young people
    HIV and STI education projects, 3
    questions for situation analysis, 194
youth, social activities for, 115
Youth Participatory Development Program, 116

zidovudine, 141
Zimbabwe, 109–10

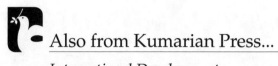 Also from Kumarian Press...

International Development

Advocacy for Social Justice: A Global Action and Reflection Guide
David Cohen, Rosa de la Vega and Gabrielle Watson

Going Global: Transforming Relief and Development NGOs
Marc Lindenberg and Coralie Bryant

Managing Policy Reform: Concepts and Tools for Decision-Makers in Developing and Transitioning Countries
Derick W. Brinkerhoff and Benjamin L. Crosby

Patronage or Partnership: Local Capacity Building in Humanitarian Crises
Edited by Ian Smillie for the Humanitarianism and War Project

Conflict Resolution, Environment, Gender Studies, Global Issues, Globalization, Microfinance, Political Economy

Bringing the Food Economy Home: Local Alternatives to Global Agribusiness
Helena Norberg-Hodge, Todd Merrifield and Steven Gorelick

The Commercialization of Microfinance
Balancing Business and Development
Edited by Deborah Drake and Elisabeth Rhyne

The Humanitarian Enterprise: Dilemmas and Discoveries
Larry Minear

Managing Drug Supply: The Selection, Procurement, Distribution, and Use of Pharmaceuticals, SECOND EDITION
Management Sciences for Health in collaboration with the World Health Organization

Pathways Out of Poverty: Innovations in Microfinance for the Poorest Families
Edited by Sam Daley-Harris

Running Out of Control: Dilemmas of Globalization
R. Alan Hedley

Shifting Burdens: Gender and Agrarian Change under Neoliberalism
Edited by Shahra Razavi

War's Offensive on Women
The Humanitarian Challenge in Bosnia, Kosovo and Afghanistan
Julie A. Mertus for the Humanitarianism and War Project

Where Corruption Lives
Edited by Gerald E. Caiden, O.P. Dwivedi and Joseph Jabbra

Visit Kumarian Press at **www.kpbooks.com** or
call **toll-free 800.289.2664** for a complete catalog.

Kumarian Press, located in Bloomfield, Connecticut, is a forward-looking, scholarly press that promotes active international engagement and an awareness of global connectedness.